The Best ORAL SEX Ever

Her Guide to Going Down

The Best ORAL SEX Ever

Her Guide to Going Down

Yvonne K. Fulbright, PhD

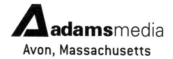

Avon, Massachusetts

Published by
Adams Media, a division of F+W Media, Inc.
57 Littlefield Street, Avon, MA 02322. U.S.A.
www.adamsmedia.com

ISBN 10: 1-4405-1076-8
ISBN 13: 978-1-4405-1076-2
eISBN 10: 1-4405-1134-9
eISBN 13: 978-1-4405-1134-9

Printed in the United States of America.

10 9 8 7 6 5 4 3 2 1

Library of Congress Cataloging-in-Publication Data
Fulbright, Yvonne K.
The best oral sex ever : her guide to going down / Yvonne K. Fulbright.
p. cm.
Includes index.
ISBN-13: 978-1-4405-1076-2
ISBN-10: 1-4405-1076-8
ISBN-13: 978-1-4405-1134-9 (ebook)
ISBN-10: 1-4405-1134-9 (ebook)
1. Oral sex. 2. Sex instruction for women. I. Title.
HQ31.5.O73F85 2011
613.9'6—dc22
2010038957

This publication is designed to provide accurate and authoritative information with
regard to the subject matter covered. It is sold with the understanding that the pub-
lisher is not engaged in rendering legal, accounting, or other professional advice. If
legal advice or other expert assistance is required, the services of a competent professional person should be sought.
—From a *Declaration of Principles* jointly adopted by a Committee of the American
Bar Association and a Committee of Publishers and Associations

Many of the designations used by manufacturers and sellers to distinguish their product
are claimed as trademarks. Where those designations appear in this book and Adams
Media was aware of a trademark claim, the designations have been printed with initial
capital letters.

Illustrations © Eric Andrews
Interior photographs credit FotoSearch/Image Source

This book is available at quantity discounts for bulk purchases.
For information, please call 1-800-289-0963.

To all of my dedicated readers—your interest and enthusiasm in all of my work mean so much!

ACKNOWLEDGMENTS

Thanks to Katie Corcoran Lytle and Katrina Schroeder, and everyone else on the Adams Media team, for their guidance and feedback. It's always a pleasure to write books for you guys!

My deepest thanks to my amazing family and friends for their never-ending support and encouragement in all that I do: Charles G. Fulbright, Ósk Lárusdóttir Fulbright, Xavier Þór Fulbright, Lauren Fulbright, Rick Barth, Solveig Bergh, Lymaraina D'Souza, Sean Duffy, Tiffany J. Franklin, Bianca A. Grimaldi, Cheri Heathscott, Marci Hunn, Jenn Kilgus, and Ásgeir Sigfússon—plus everyone at home in Iceland! It has been a breathtaking year of travel, opportunity, growth, and change—and I couldn't have done it without you. xoxo

Contents

INTRODUCTION
Open Up and Say "Ahhhh . . . "

If you've cracked open this book, your curiosity has been piqued. Oral sex has a way of doing that, beckoning lovers to come get a taste. Those who have been there know it's *the* means to better, more fulfilling orgasms. Those who haven't gone down under—or those who have been disappointed by earlier experiences—at least know its reputation for inviting sexual release in a way that nothing else can. There's no doubt that going down on your partner has taken center stage in the quest for sexual fulfillment. It seems like everyone wants more than a mouthful, and who can blame them?

Becoming an oral connoisseur is where it's at when it comes to reaching new, jaw-dropping sexual heights. However, while your aim is to give him the best head ever, this book is very much about how to make the experience of giver the best for you too. After all, a pleasure shared is a pleasure doubled, and your ability to not only deliver the most effective techniques around, but love what you're doing, while you're doing it, is critical to both your and your partner's erotic experience.

The Best Oral Sex Ever: Her Guide to Going Down is intended for lovers looking for erotic ideas, couples hoping to deal with their oral sex issues, and women seeking to make oral sex more palpable or more of a priority in their passion pursuits. It will answer all of those questions that you're too afraid or too embarrassed to ask. As with any sex act, oral sex mastery comes with time, dedication, practice, and desire and, as a sex educator and relationship expert, I know well the trials and tribulations that lovers grapple with when it comes to fellatio. Fortunately, this book will send you well on your way, offering oral sex tips and techniques, and strategies to help you overcome any barriers, as well as:

- A whole new level of "sexpertise."
- Realistic erotic expectations.
- How to communicate your needs, concerns, and questions to your partner.
- The information and skills needed to take care of both your and your partner's sexual health while doing what you'll learn to do best.
- Tons of instruction on how to eroticize oral sex and how to get both you and your partner off.
- Information on his potential for multiple orgasms.
- Referrals you can turn to for more information.

I can't say it enough—going down on your guy can offer some of the greatest pleasures and most intimate moments that you'll ever experience. The confidence and power trip that comes with knowing that you're an expert at giving head is an ego boost like no other. By the end of this book, you'll be on top of your game, feeling great about your ability to help him feel more than a little sexually satisfied.

As you read through the following pages, it's important to remember that sexual preferences are as numerous as there are people. How to make oral sex an art form for *your* sexual partner needs to be explored and you'll need to specially tailor your skills to his wants and likes. Some things may work after one or many tries; others may not. Some techniques may work at another stage in your relationship—or with a totally different guy. If you're in your current relationship for the long-haul, you'll want to come back to this book more than once to keep your oral intimacy original and red hot. After all, we all evolve as lovers in our pleasures, reactions, and abilities.

But, no matter your experience, this book will help you to see oral sex in a whole new, healthy, exciting light. Trust me, you'll soon be delivering like an oral sex pro.

CHAPTER 1

Our Intrigue with Oral Sex

Lip service, *going down*, *sucking cock*, *giving a hummer*, *meeting with the one-eyed purple monster*. . . . The slang terms for oral sex are very creative, often quite comical, and, at the very least, many. Google "oral sex" and 17.4 million hits come up for that term alone. People around the world are intrigued with the eroticism involved in giving the genitals a slip of the tongue and more. To say we're orally fixated is an understatement.

Just So We're on the Same Page . . .

Performing oral sex is a universal sexual experience enjoyed by millions as a part of foreplay, as a part of afterplay (that lovely, intimate, coming down period following sexual intercourse), or as the main sex event. In those racy trysts involving more than two sexual partners, it can even be experienced during sexual intercourse. In any case, oral-genital contact, more commonly known as *oral sex*, involves giving or receiving pleasure delivered to a person's sexual organs primarily via the lips and tongue. This is typically done in a rhythmic licking or sucking fashion using one's mouth, though any number of techniques can be employed, as we'll cover in-depth throughout this book.

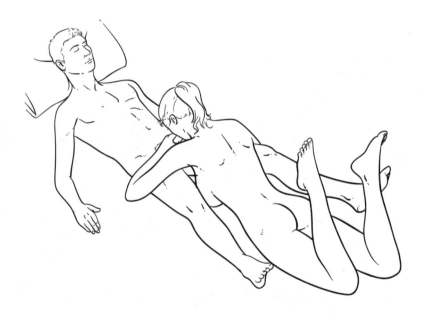

Stemming from the Latin *fellare*, which literally means "to suck," *fellatio* is the formal term for oral stimulation of the male penis and scrotum—aka *blow job* or *giving head*. Another form of oral sex, *analingus*—also known as *rimming, ass licking, eating ass,* or *tossing salad*—refers to oral-anal contact. Anal-oral sex may accompany fellatio or may be the sole event of a sex session. Now while this may sound somewhat technical, these types of sexual exchanges can be quite titillating. Sucking cock is a highly effective erotic technique, which has held rapture for humans throughout the ages. Analingus, which we'll cover here and there throughout this book, is more of an acquired taste, but something that really works for couples who are into it. Whether sought for its scintillating sensations, or pursued as a prime opportunity to get down and dirty, any of these oral adventures is the favorite kind of sex to be had for a number of lovers for a number of reasons.

| Why He Loves Oral Sex

In choosing your oral sex seductions and strategies, it's best to start by getting in his head. What is it about blow jobs that guys love so much? Obviously, he loves the feel-good sensations that can only come from oral sex. He loves that the mouth is wet, warm, and soft, and that it can tighten around his shaft while skillfully hitting all the right parts. Unbeknownst to many, though, is that men, generally, are often all about oral for psychological reasons as well. As receiver, your guy feels hero worshipped, and, along with that, desired, accepted, nurtured, and dominant. He also adores the fact that you are doing all of the work.

Rolls Off the Tongue

"Oral sex is a treat—there's nothing like it. I love having all types of other sex, but having a warm mouth wrapped around my cock is one of the most amazing sensations ever. And the fact that I don't have to do anything, but enjoy, makes it only better." } Naveen

Pleasure from Power

The ego trip your partner may receive when getting head can be intoxicating for him. Being the object of your devotion only adds to the adoration he has for oral. With his dream or fantasy lover between his legs, how can he help but not get caught up in the high of being pleasured? Your guy only gets hotter when he glances down at what's going on between his legs; the mere visual stimulation that comes from seeing (and imagining in his off-time) your head bobbing around can be highly arousing.

Of course, let's not forget the power trip in this exchange for you, and the elation that comes along with being giver. While the giver is often cast in a submissive role, in actuality, that's not the case. You're the partner in charge, which can set fire to your inner dominatrix. In getting the green light to go down, you've been granted V.I.P. access to your partner's prime hot spots. His pleasure is in your hands. You control your man's sexual destiny (at least for the moment) by commanding the action—all with the best seat in the house.

Sex Savvy

Despite its mass popularity, believe it or not, oral sex is on the books as illegal in some states, like Indiana—even when consensual and with another adult. So for those of you dead set on breaking the law, let this bad-ass bit fuel hotter oral. After all, such restrictions and concerns have helped to fetishize oral sex over the ages. Because it's often considered taboo in nature, oral sex occupies a great deal of people's fantasies. So for those of you who can legally have fellatio, stoke the same thrills by pretending you're doing it in Indiana.

So don't be afraid to let yourself get turned on by seeing your man become sexually excited, an experience made even sweeter when the object of your affection hits heaven. He may not be in that alone. As giver, you can thrive on your own "mental orgasm" in knowing that he is thoroughly enjoying your efforts. You created the moment necessary for sexual release, and that can be incredibly fulfilling.

Popular Culture: The Oral Sex Buzz

These days it feels like oral sex is everywhere. The attention contemporary lovers give oral action—and the attention givers are expected to give it—is greatly influenced by the massive media exposure oral fixations have received. You can credit the porn industry for making fellatio the main feature in a number of triple-X rated movies, the most popular of which continues to be the 1972's *Deep Throat*, featuring porn star Linda Lovelace. Lovelace plays a sexually frustrated woman on a mission to realize her first orgasm. A doctor incorrectly tells her that her clitoris is located in the back of her throat, inspiring Lovelace to perform oral sex on various men.

Yet for all of *Deep Throat*'s popularity, oral endeavors remained largely under the public's radar until the infamous Bill Clinton/Monica Lewinsky scandal in the late nineties when then White House intern Lewinsky delivered the most famous blow job ever during President Clinton's second term in office. The controversy surrounding the sexual exchange ultimately made oral sex everyday conversation, and, some would argue, a more everyday event.

Mainstream pop culture films since both *Deep Throat* and the Clinton scandal have regularly involved scenes suggesting oral activity, with main characters in movies like 1997's *Chasing Amy* discussing blow job techniques as easily and commonly as they would talk about the weather. The music industry, too, has gotten in on the act over the years, portraying oral sex positively, and perhaps influencing public perceptions of such pleasuring for the better.

In the late 1980s, Madonna hinted at assuming position for head in "Like a Prayer" with "I'm down on my knees. I wanna take you there." In the early nineties, Liz Phair murmured her desire to be a "blow job queen" with lyrics that stated, "Your dick's a perfect suck me size" in "Flower." In more recent years, a number of the songs on oral sex have come from the hip-hop/R&B music genre from singers like Prince, Lil Kim, and Khia. In "Just Put It in Your Mouth," Akinyele aggressively (and arguably offensively) commands the action with " . . . you can lick it, you can flip it, you can taste it. I'm talking every drip-drop, don't waste it." With the ultimate in oral sex tips a regular headliner and feature in online and hardcopy media outlets alike, oral sex inspirations are even showing up in the publishing industry in books and magazines.

This eagerness for anything oral has, however, perpetuated some of the myths and misconceptions tackled in this book. For example, while women's magazines tend to treat oral sex traditionally, as something done to enhance relationship intimacy, men's magazines tend to detach it from the relationship. For guys, oral sex is cast as an experience in and of itself, requiring none of the excuses or symbolism it supposedly does for a woman. While there is some truth in some generalities, buyer beware! In enjoying such articles, you need to be mindful about the messages you're getting about oral sex, recognizing how the media may be influencing your thoughts and practices around such pleasuring.

Rolls Off the Tongue

"My wife went down on me at my best friend's wedding reception in a changing room. It was *hot*. We were both liquored up in celebration, and she grabbed me firmly and demanded that I let her give it to me (she's not a big sexual aggressor so it made it even more hot). Naturally, I was in." }Johann

Oral Sex Today

Despite our growing acceptance of oral sex, it still regularly poses controversy. As recently as 2010, dictionaries were removed from southern California classrooms after a parent complained that a child could read the definition for the term *oral sex*. The school district responded by pulling Merriam Webster's 10th edition from shelves for fear that it was too "sexually graphic" and inappropriate for certain age groups. Still, despite regularly ruffling feathers, oral sex has become increasingly frequent, regarded more and more as an important and healthy component of one's sexual self.

While not as widely practiced as other types of sexual behaviors, like vaginal-penile intercourse, oral sex is a very common practice. If any hesitancy you have in engaging in oral comes down to safety in numbers, rest assured. Various studies show that such sexual behaviors are practiced by the majority of people, with about 90 percent of men and women ages twenty-five to forty-four reporting having ever engaged in oral sex. People of all orientations and ages, including adolescents and the elderly, engage in oral pleasuring.

Sex Savvy

She didn't! She did. According to Kitty Kelley's biography of Nancy Reagan, *Nancy Reagan: The Unauthorized Biography*, the former First Lady was known in Hollywood for giving the best blow job in town during her days as actress Nancy Davis. "Just-say-yes Nancy," as she was called, was apparently quite popular on the MGM lot for her office visits and evening rendezvous.

Oral Sex Attitudes

On a cultural level, Americans have been assessing just how *laissez-faire* they've gotten, in general, about going down on strangers and regular lovers alike. People of the Baby Boomer generation recall oral sex as having been saved for the most intimate of sexual relationships, creating a type of special bond between lovers when at long last explored. For women, in particular, giving head was somehow a bigger deal than sexual intercourse, and regarded as a privilege of being intimate in a loving, nonexploitative, long-term union. Reciprocity was also a big part of her willingness to give. If she went down on her male lover, it was expected that he would do the same.

This guarded attitude towards fellatio was largely based on social notions at the time, namely, that giving head reduced a woman to no more than a subordinate—as in literally on her hands and knees—servicing agent. Swallowing only reinforced that she was being dominated, something her inner feminist could only allow to a point. This one-way depiction of oral sex has withstood the test of time in modern society's worship of the alpha male and its desire to fuel his next power trip with sex that's all about his pleasuring. This one-sided pleasuring is seen in porn, glorifying male sexual pursuits, conquests, and satisfaction, more than anywhere else. Being made to feel like a servicing agent, porn star, or simply disrespected is part of what can hold back a number of men's lovers. On the other hand, some women, including feminists, feel that embracing the triple-X quality of oral sex is empowering, super pleasurable, and hotter, whether hooking up with an alpha male or not.

Sociologists have suggested that oral sex has become less about intimacy in the decades since the sexual revolution, with lovers focusing less on the emotional bond and more on technique and competence. Some point to Monica Lewinsky's oral antics as the makings of the current overall oral sex superficiality in America. Her overly analyzed blow job wasn't about making love or a symbol of commitment and giving of one's self. It was seen as something practically everyday and shallow, judgments easily reinforced in that the act became something that she eventually made money off of. Contrast this handling of oral sex with other cultures, like the French, where oral sex isn't taken so lightly. French author Thierry Leguay, who wrote *The History of Fellatio* (currently only available in French), has argued that "You'll never find a French Monica Lewinsky." For the French, generally speaking, oral sex is an act with a lot more meaning.

Sex Q & A

Are humans the only species on earth that engage in oral sex?

Yes, many animals may engage in oral-genital stimulation, especially when the female is in estrue (heat). While it's more of a play behavior for juvenile male bonobos, the fruit bat licks her mate's penis during copulation. She does this by lowering her head to lick his shaft or the base of his penis while the glans of the penis is still in her vagina—and all while in a "hanging position." Interestingly enough, the male never withdraws his penis when it's being licked, extending the length of time spent copulating. Mother Nature is such a genius sometimes.

Degree of Intimacy

Oral sex can be a very personal, intimate sexual experience for some people and no big deal to others. For some people, oral exchanges are reserved for partners whom they feel really close to, whereas for others, it's a staple part of every sexual affair handled with indifference. Some regard oral intimacies as a marker of how lovers feel about each other sexually and emotionally, making a relationship all the more exclusive. Others see oral trysts as no more than a cheap thrill, as is the case with "glory holes," where a man places his penis in the hole of a public bathroom wall for totally anonymous head. In a number of cases, the degree of intimacy can come down to the situation and the person to whom you're giving head.

Rolls Off the Tongue

"Honestly, the only times I enjoy it is in nightclub stalls with random people. And I don't even enjoy it physically (except maybe once); it's nothing more than an ego boost." } Adam

But, casual or not, having oral sex is quite physically intimate for both the giver and receiver. In most giving scenarios, your face is up close and personal with your lover's groin and thighs. Beyond the meaning some place on this act, being up close and personal can in and of itself make the experience extremely emotionally intimate. In fact, for some, oral sex is more intimate than intercourse since it involves your head and face. In addition, symbolically, oral sex is the meeting of the cultured, reasoning, intellectual (top) half of one's self with what's regarded as another's raw, carnal, unrefined (bottom) half. The impermissible nature of this meeting violates social order. A sense of intimacy—and libidinal energy—is practically immediate in lovers daring to defy social taboos together. Sure does cast Romeo and Juliet's longings in a whole new light, no?

| The Importance of Oral Sex

Regardless of the type of relationship you're in (or not), or the circumstances around its occurrence, *oral sex* has come to mean *hot sex*. It is a self-esteem booster to get some or give some. Oral sex can make or break a specific sex session. It can heavily influence the quality of a couple's sex life for the better, when regularly engaged in, or for the worse, when given zero attention. This very intimate form of connection can be a relationship strengthener, with many men taking it quite personally when their partners want nothing to do with going down on them.

Rolls Off the Tongue

"When I was in high school, my Dad was driving my girlfriend and I home from a ski trip. We were in the back seat, and my girlfriend started giving me a blow job with my Dad two feet away until it got too noisy. Then she finished with her hand. It was so good in part because she was so good at it, but in particular, because I was so surprised." } Brad

Oral sex is the best kind of sex for some people, with many holding that it is unlike anything else. This sexy gift of pleasure offers excitement, variety, exhilaration, and closeness. Many men adore the more precise targeting of erogenous zones that comes with oral sex, often feeling heightened sensitivity as their lover makes them moan. Your tongue and lips feel amazing against your lover's sensitive genitals; many men even liken a hot, wet mouth to the inside of a nice, tight vagina. Oral sex can even be meditative, with your partner slipping into a zen-like state of enlightenment in reaching a heightened state of awareness that can be spiritual in nature.

This reaching bliss bit starts with knowing the ins and outs of his genitals. In Chapter 2, we send you well on your way to delivering the best ever by going over the basics of his external and internal sexual anatomy. There's more to his member than meets the eye, and it's all about to meet your tongue.

Sexual Anatomy: Passion-Inducing Parts

Before you can become a blow-job connoisseur, you need to know exactly what you're working with. I'm sure you already know that a penis and scrotum are a big (maybe even huge?) part of his crown jewels, but do you really know which exact parts are best to target when you get down there? While his pride and joy is very much an erogenous zone in and of itself, there is so much more to explore. Whether you're bringing your partner's penis to life or maximizing his pleasure once he's at attention, you'll want to spend some time becoming well acquainted with his oft-overlooked, but most reactive hot spots. Prepare to see his penis in a whole new light as we talk about what else there is to explore down under to make sure your mouth moves are even more magnificent.

Learn Your Way Around the Landscape

While some people are lucky enough to cover the anatomy of sex at some point in their schooling, the vast majority never thoroughly learn about the ins and outs of some of our most amazing private parts! The result: Many lovers have no clue what is where, how to play with a juicy bit, or how to reach peak sexual response with spots that are solely for pleasure. Not your average biology lesson, the following sections on his genitalia are among the most important in this book if your aim is to become a better, savvier lover. Here, you get the quick 'n' dirty low down on your lover's sexual makeup. If you get confused, check out the following image.

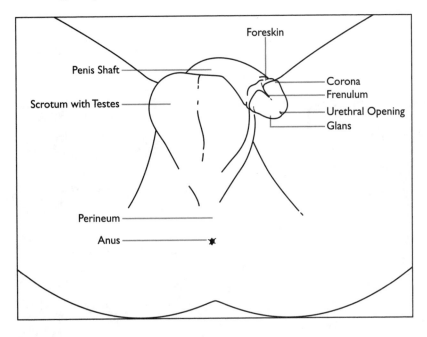

Pinpoint His Outer Hot Spots

Do a quick scan of a male's groin area and you'll notice that it consists of the penis and scrotum. Yet a more thorough investigation of the individual erogenous zones sprinkled all over this area would reveal the following:

Glans. The "head" of the penis, the glans is the smooth, very sensitive helmet-shaped knob at the tip. Chock full of nerve endings, it has the potential to send tremors throughout your lover's body when aptly attended to.

Foreskin. Most males around the world are intact or uncircumcised—meaning the foreskin of their penis hasn't been removed. Their lovers have the wonders of an additional erotic area to awaken since this retractable, double-layered fold of skin is packed full of rich blood vessels, nerve endings, and muscle fibers. (Note: Males who are circumcised have had this erogenous tissue removed.)

Urethral Opening. The slit-like opening of the glans, through which urine, pre-ejaculate, and semen pass, is the urethral opening. Since it's filled with nerve endings, some men find stimulation of this area quite arousing, though many find it painful or uncomfortable. Proceed with caution!

Shaft. This body of the penis, covered with muscles (but not a muscle itself), is filled with blood vessels and contains spongy cylinders—a pair of *corpora cavernosa* and a *corpus spongiosum*—that fill with blood when your lover is aroused, expanding and causing an erection. This area can handle a lot more stimulation than the smaller, more delicate erogenous zones can individually, in part because the *corpora cavernosa* extends back into a man's body, with its *crural* (roots) attaching to branches of the pelvis. This prevents his penis from sinking into his body during thrusting. As many men will tell you, they can handle a lot more than what most lovers assume. So don't be shy in taking charge!

Corona. No, we're not talking beer here. The *corona* or *coronal ridge* is the raised ridge at the bottom of the glans that separates the shaft from the head of the penis. This is the most excitable region for some guys. Easier to find on guys who have been circumcised, the corona is best identified on an uncircumcised man once he's fully erect.

Frenulum. The *frenulum* or *fraenum* is found on the underside of the penis, where the shaft and head of the penis meet. This small bump of loose skin is extremely sensitive, and may appear as an area of scar tissue in males who have been circumcised. In some men, this bump is the most sensitive part of the penis, so be careful! Your lover can reach the finish line too quickly if the stimulation you deliver is overly intense.

Scrotum. The dark, thick-skinned sac of very sensitive flesh hanging between a male's legs, the *scrotum*—more commonly known as the *balls*—houses your man's testicles. When a guy gets cold, the muscles of his scrotal sac contract, drawing the testicles closer to the body and causing slight shrinkage. These muscles also relax when he's hot, lowering the testicles away from the body in an effort to maintain the ideal temperature for sperm production. While it's tempting to roughhouse with your lover's balls, the area should be handled with care, unless he tells you he can handle more; the sensitivity of this area varies from guy to guy.

Rolls Off the Tongue

"In some ways, I have more fun with scrotal play than anything else during oral. I think it's because this area is so sensitive and soft and feels so nice in my mouth. His scent can also be highly arousing, which I've found is more the case if I'm really into a guy." } Chanel

Perineum. Not all of your lover's erogenous zones are found on his penis. If you move up to the area between where his balls meets his body and the anus, you'll find the perineum—an area of soft tissue and nerve endings. This is a major hot spot for a number of men, in part because stimulation of this area indirectly brings his highly erogenous prostate to life (see a description of the prostate below). While a challenge to stimulate orally, manually toying with this area while sucking on your guy's lollipop can enhance your oral efforts.

Pinpoint His Inner Hot Spots

A male's internal reproductive system includes the *testis, epididymis, vas deferens, bulbourethral gland, Cowper's gland,* and *prostate.* Two of these areas are worth homing in on during oral, depending on your guy's preferences:

Testicles. Also referred to as the *testes* or *gonads,* your guy's testicles are indirectly stimulated when you play with his balls, which protect them. These oval glands are critical to a man's pleasure on the most basic level because they produce sex hormones, primarily testosterone, which influence his sex drive as well as his sperm. Testicles vary in size and shape, with the left testicle typically hanging lower than the right one—supposedly so that they don't bang into one another. One testicle may also be slightly larger than the other.

Prostate. Fondly referred to as the *P-spot,* the prostate surrounds the urethra, sitting just below the bladder above the perineum. When a guy is sexually excited, this firm, golf ball–sized gland of smooth muscle fibers, connective tissues, small tubes, clusters of glands, and tiny blood vessels throbs, sending sensations throughout his pelvic region as it swells with prostatic fluid, which seeks to protect the sperm from the vagina's acidity, helping sperm movement and improving the chance of fertilization. Some guys dig prostate stimulation, which is easily done by massaging your first two knuckles up against his perineum, and are blown away by the incredible way its reactions rock their world; others feel that it does nothing for their sexual response and others find it downright uncomfortable. Your lover's feelings about prostate play actually can change from one sex session to the next, underscoring the need to find out what he fancies each time you go down on him.

| What Happens When He Gets Hot 'n' Horny

First researched and outlined by sexologists in the 1960s, the "sexual response cycle" involves a general pattern of events that the majority of people experience when they get turned on. There are five phases:

- Desire.
- Arousal.
- Plateau.
- Orgasm.
- Resolution.

While these stages generally happen in sequence, your lover (or you) can experience these responses in any order. He may also "stray" off of this beaten path, with his body doing what works for him. The blueprint for sexual response varies from guy to guy and from time to time, and is influenced by a number of factors. That said, let's take a closer look at these stages and what you can expect during each one.

Desire

An entity of its own, separate from sexual arousal, desire motivates us to take actions into our own hands so to speak. It urges us to seek out a partner, pursue sexual opportunities, engage in sexual behaviors, and get our rocks off. Desire can be sparked, intentionally or not, by sex objects, physical arousal, fantasies, spontaneous excitement, longings, images, sounds, scents, memories, interests, or experiences—any of which can be sensual, pornographic, thrilling, or heart-soaring. Desire can come on unexpectedly or you or your lover may actively seek it out. It is impacted by health, mood, and attitudes, among a whole host of biological, psychological, and social factors.

Sex Savvy

It's a true chicken-or-the-egg debate: Does desire really come before arousal or is it the other way around? Some sexologists are now saying that desire doesn't always have to come first; it may be a reaction we have to a subliminal or physical sensation, like touch. In other words, your body and his appear to be primed for sex!

Arousal

During this phase, your body prepares itself for sex. You're likely to notice faster, heavier breathing, an accelerated heart rate, a sex flush (a reddening of the chest, neck, and sometimes face), and/or lubrication. This is in large part because the body is experiencing muscle tension (*myotonia*) and, the accumulation of blood in the genitals (*vasocongestion*), which causes them to become harder, darker, more swollen; the skin of your partner's balls will thicken now as well. This is also the time when your guy's erection will appear, in addition to a slight elevation of his scrotum.

Plateau

A state of high arousal, this phase extends heightened sexual response. You and your lover may experience a continued sex flush, faster breathing, and a higher blood pressure and heart rate. You may even experience short muscle spasms in your face, hands, and feet. At this point, your lover will have a full erection; his penis will darken in color and the tip will swell. His balls will be even more swollen, and will have risen even higher. Pre-cum may also have made its way out of the tip of the penis, leaving the passageway clean and clear for sperm.

Orgasm

As I'm sure you know, orgasm involves an intense series of rhythmic pelvic and muscle contractions as the body releases sexual tension. Your and your lover's pulse rates, breathing, blood pressure, and sex flushes will be at their highest levels. For a guy, ejaculation almost always accompanies climax because the muscles at the root of his penis and the urethral bulb will force semen out of his urethral opening while he finishes.

Sex Q & A

Is orgasm necessary for sexual satisfaction?

While climax is often seen as the *crème de la crème* of sexual response, it isn't vital to sexual gratification. A number of men and women have reported that sex without orgasm can be very satisfying, in part because they value the other oh-so-sexy components involved in ideal sex, including being in-sync with their partners, erotic intimacy, connectedness, and being present and uninhibited.

Resolution

In this final phase of the sexual response cycle, lovers come down from heightened arousal. Here, men lose their erection in two stages. First, blood leaves the penis, though it will remain slightly larger and more sensitive than normal for a bit. Second, a refractory period sets in, during which time your guy will not physically be able to get hard or get off.

Again, remember that this is a loose road map for a lot of people, so don't get hung up on what's going on (or not) when. Get caught up in what's going on in the moment—the sexual energy exchange and the fun you and your partner are having pursuing a shared pleasure; all of that is what pushes everything else over the top.

Rolls Off the Tongue

"Some of the best ever that I've had was from a girl who enjoyed giving! She would lube my entire dick with her saliva and then use her hand and her mouth in the most amazing coordinated effort I've ever experienced. She seemed to find the same amount of satisfaction in my orgasm as I did." } Gary

| Meet Your Tongue

It's all too easy to dive into what's below-the-belt when charting your sexual pleasure pursuits. But when it comes to oral sex, it's not a bad idea to examine the muscular organ of the mouth in addition to the pelvic area's playground. Your tongue can very well be considered a sexual organ in its own right. It's not only one of the main sources of exhilaration for a receiver, it plays a major role in your pleasure as well—and in ways that are often neglected. So let's explore the ways that this little-understood love muscle enhances oral sex:

Movement. The tongue can move in almost every direction, as well as compress and expand. It enables you to manipulate your guy's business with up-down, side-to-side, and in-and-out motions, and with great skill and exact pressure.

Texture. Coated with a moist, pink tissue known as *mucosa*, the tongue is covered with tiny bumps called *papillae* that give it its rough texture. These bumps create the friction that adds to your partner's pleasure.

Taste. The papillae are covered with thousands of taste buds, which are collections of nerve-like cells that connect to the brain via nerve pathways. Each contains 50–150 taste receptor cells for detecting the chemical makeup of solutions, enabling you to detect if your lover's genitals or fluids are sweet, salty, bitter, sour (acid), umami (savory), and/or fatty. The flavor of your feast is a combination of taste, smell, touch, temperature, and consistency (texture).

Sex Savvy

Stephen Taylor of the U.K. holds the Guinness World Record for longest tongue, measuring at 3.74 inches beyond the center of his closed top lip.

Feel. Your tongue is sensitive to temperature and texture, which help you to analyze all of those other qualities that add to your pleasures, like the groin's density, oiliness, texture, and *viscosity* (consistency).

Moisture. The tongue is covered by a double-layered mucous membrane, the *epithelial* (surface) layer of which secretes mucus to moisten your mouth and whatever you're munching on.

It may seem a little silly to point out these characteristics until you consider just how little attention these qualities of the tongue are given. While food and wine connoisseurs give a great deal of thought to their palates—and what's going on in the mouth—even the best of oral sex enthusiasts don't give a second thought to what their tongue is truly experiencing beyond initial taste and texture perceptions. Yet tuning into the texture, taste, feel, and moisture components of giving and receiving oral sex can heighten the eroticism involved, putting lovers fully in tune with their sexual responses and the sex act itself. Don't deprive yourself of experiencing oral to its fullest!

Rolls Off the Tongue

"It's so easy to get caught up in what I'm doing, namely technique, when I provide pleasuring. But when you tune into what your tongue is experiencing, you start to notice subtleties in the action—and reactions I'm having—which makes for a richer, and tastier, experience." } Elaina

Now that you know all about the naughty parts to play with, we're going to get to the info you've been most eagerly awaiting: info on positions. Oral sex can be had in many different ways, and comes down to what one or both of you wants—or perhaps what the situation calls for. In expanding your sexual repertoire and changing things up on occasion, Chapter 3 will have you reconsidering your approach and, much to his delight, all of the places you could possibly assume the position.

Naked Twister Gets Naughty: Positions for Oral Sex

Naked Twister takes on a totally new meaning when you approach traditional sexual positions with oral sex in mind. How you lay, stand, bend, angle, and so on, influences the sensations you receive or deliver, and how easily your guy can relish the sensations meant solely for him. This may or may not involve employing erotic furniture and supports. While some positions are ideal for peak performance, others are pursued simply for the variety, for shaking up your routine, and others are meant to amp up excitement in their novelty or exotic nature.

NOTE: Just so we're not faulted for not stating it: Some of these positions may require a great deal of athleticism, strength, and/or flexibility. While exciting and enticing, don't push the limits on what you or your partner is capable of; winding up in the ER with a sex injury is anything but hot!

| The Classic

Why couples love it: This relaxing, comfortable position offers you all access to his groin, making penetration of his anus easy—if that's what he likes, of course.

Him: The classic lets your lover take a load off as he gets to lay back and relax as you go to town. Having him propped up on pillows is optional, but ideal in helping him to visually enjoy your porn-star performance.

You: While you can kneel between your lover's thighs, it's easier to lie down on your stomach, your arms wrapped under your lover's thighs for better leverage, support, control, and stimulation. Another way to approach him is by lying down in a position perpendicular to his body.

Tips:

- Place a pillow under his butt for a better angle and greater comfort.
- Grasp and lift his butt as you cast your spells.
- Take action off the bed, trying other flat surfaces for the classic, like your back yard or sofa.
- Sit on his legs for a nice dominatix, pin down effect.

Variations:

- Raise one or both of his legs over your shoulder(s).
- Bend either or both of his legs into his chest.
- Prop his feet on your shoulders.
- Have his legs splayed or close together.

- Instead of facing him, position yourself so you're looking the other way.
- Sit on his chest for an almost 69.
- For more direct anal play, have him lift his legs completely over your head.
- Scoot him to the edge of the bed so that his legs dangle over the side.

Rolls Off the Tongue

"This one is my favorite since all I need to do is lay back and relax. It's the perfect way to end a tough day or get sent off to sleep." } Matt

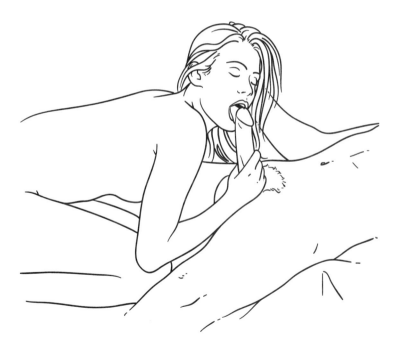

Starfish

Why couples love it: Anything exotic is automatically sexy.

Him: Have him lie on his back, with his legs spread.

You: Lie on your stomach, between your lover's legs.

Tips: "Torture" your lover by keeping his legs spread while the action becomes more heated. Do this by pressing down on the knees or calves and playing with the back of his knees—the location of a sexual reflexology point. This point, called *San-Yin-Chiao*, is inside of the shin, approximately three inches above the anklebone and beside the shinbone; it's a place where three energy channels intersect.

On Your Knees

Why couples love it: What guy doesn't like it when his girl looks like she's begging to attend to his every oral need?? It plays into his, at least occasional, desire to be dominant. Your guy will think it's incredibly hot to see his penis disappearing into your mouth. Additionally, this position is great for both of you if you're looking for a quickie.

Him: He may want to lean against a firm support, like a couch or wall, for comfort and for better balance.

You: Kneel in front of your lover, resting your knees on a pillow, cushion, or folded blanket or towel so that this position isn't too hard on your knees.

Tips: Grip his hips and bum. This enables you to take him deeper into your mouth when pleasuring him. Consider springing this position on him the next time you undress him!

Variations:

- Have him prop one of his legs up on a support for greater control as he stands.
- Have him face away from you and stick out his butt for better access in coming from behind his body.

- Have him bend over to show off his full moon for even greater access.

Rolls Off the Tongue

"I feel guilty saying it since I respect women, but there's a head trip that comes along with having a babe on her knees with your cock in her mouth. I get a slight rush of power that makes me want her more." }

Cole

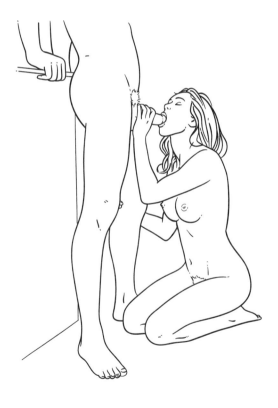

Sitting

Why couples love it: So many sitting surfaces of various heights to choose from! Plus, this position can be easier on your neck. Your partner will love that he gets to see you between his legs, and that it's easy for you to get so many strokes in.

Him: Have your lover sit in the chair of choice—barstool, armchair, recliner, kitchen table chair, and so on, and have him hook his ankles around the front two legs or over the arms for easier access.

You: Your lover's height on the chair (plus the length of your own body) will determine if you need to go at this one kneeling, sitting on the floor, squatting, or standing.

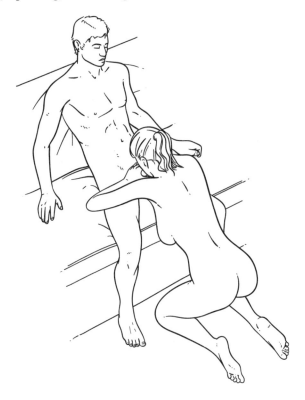

Tips: Ask him to show you some appreciation by delivering a loving head massage as you work away. He can also cup the back of your head to encourage more vigorous or deeper action when desired, if you like that type of guidance.

Variations: Don't limit yourself to traditional chairs. Make use of anywhere your lover can sit, like your dining room table, kitchen counter, the stairs, the edge of the bed, or on your car's back seat. Up for a real challenge? Have him assume a squatting position.

| Face-Sitting

Why couples love it: With this position, your guy takes charge by sliding his penis across your tongue and mouth. This is ideal if you like full-on oral contact with his genitals and anus.

Him: Have your lover straddle you, placing his knees on either side of your chest before sitting on it. To make this position as comfortable as possible, have him lean forward. Remind him that he can lower his body for more pressure against his jewels or elevate himself more for less stimulation.

You: In this position, you are on your back with your lover straddling your face; he controls the pace—to a degree. All you need to do is move your head, mouth, and tongue, allowing yourself to get into it. However, be sure to let your partner know if you're feeling suffocated at any point. You'll want to have a key signal, like two taps on his thigh, to indicate that he's getting carried away with any thrusting. This action is fun until you're choking on it! Even though this is a submissive position, keep in mind that you're ultimately the one in charge.

Tips: He can prop himself up against a wall or a bed's headboard for more support and better balance and you can grip your lover's buttocks to better control his thrusts. You can also prop yourself up slightly with pillows for easier action.

Variations:

- Have your lover hover over you instead of pulling a face plant.
- Change directions, meaning have him sit the other way in riding your face, especially if you want deeper tongue penetration of the anus. If you bend your legs, he can rest against your knees for support if desired.
- If he's tall enough, ask him to stand at the edge of the bed while sitting on your face.
- He can squat instead of kneel, but this probably won't be as comfortable for him, and may pose the risk of him falling on you when he gets caught up in his climax.

Rolls Off the Tongue

"For some reason, I like anal play when getting head sometimes. I didn't know this until I was with my wife and she surprised me with a little. She does it some 'cuz she knows I like it now, but I'd like it a little bit more often." }Grant

| From Behind

Why couples love it: Anything rear entry is hot.

Him: Have him get down on all fours for your "tongue lashing."

You: Approach your lover's genitals from behind. If you're up for it, and your partner is into it, consider analingus while you're in the area.

Tips: Take advantage of the fact that no other position allows such great access to the perineum and dig your tongue, knuckle, fingertip, or a sex toy firmly into this hot spot with a massaging motion, to unleash the sexual energy housed here—plus stimulate his prostate!

Variations:

- You can slide underneath him and position your face under his genitals. Use your forearms to lift yourself against his body.

- Have him lean down onto his forearms to provide a better angle.

Sideways

Why couples love it: There's something about leisurely lounging around.

Him: Have your lover lie down on his side.

You: Experiment with different angles, as some will allow for more shallow action, others for deeper action.

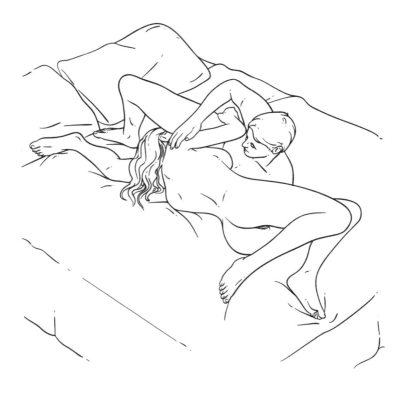

Tips: Experiment with just how far you want to part his legs, as this impacts how much you'll have to play with.

Variations:

- Both of you can be on your side.
- Approach giving head from a perpendicular angle, with your partner lying one direction across the bed and you the other. You can also have him lift his top leg for a more interesting variation with all access.

Wrap Around

Why couples love it: This oral sex position allows for amazing full body contact.

Him: All your lover has to do is sit on a couch.

You: Sit behind him and wrap yourself around his body. Now bend yourself around his side until your mouth reaches his cock. You'll ultimately end up on your side performing oral.

Tips: If you're not especially tall or flexible, consider using a cock sleeve to provide the lower half of his shaft with adequate stimulation while you focus on the head. If your hand reach isn't especially effective, don't be afraid to ask if he can, literally, lend a hand in stimulating himself.

Plough Pose

Why couples love it: What can be more perfect than the meeting of zen and bliss in assuming this inversion yoga pose, known for its relaxing, restoring effects?

Him: Have your lover lay on his back and lift his legs up straight in the air, with his hands supporting his lower back. Then have him swing his legs over his head; he may be able to touch his toes to the floor. Alternatively, he may be able to rest his knees close to his ears.

You: This position gives you more direct access to your lover than any other. Go nuts!

Tips: Check in with him periodically to make sure he's okay. Note: This position is only for guys who are flexible and physically fit (yoga experience preferred)!

Bottoms Up!

Why couples love it: His airborne genitals feel freer, and you'll have an excellent view of him thoroughly enjoying himself.

Him: Have your guy lay down and put his legs over your shoulders, as this will lift his pelvis upward.

You: Place your hands under his butt for added support, and work your magic while on your knees. In taking advantage of the angle, give ample attention to his anus and perineum, really going to town like you can't get enough.

Tips: Only attempt this if you're strong enough. If on your knees, be kind to yourself with a soft surface like pillows or a blanket.

Variations: Depending on your heights, you can try both sitting and standing while delivering.

Deep Throat

Why couples love it: Deep down, almost everybody has a Linda Lovelace fantasy that's just dying to see the light of day (or cover of night).

Him: Have your man stand beside a bed or flat surface.

You: Lie on your back, with your head hanging over the edge of the bed. Gently bend your lover's penis downward and take it into your mouth. Control the thrusting by keeping your hands on your lover's upper thighs or butt, and establishing a rhythmic pulling to set the pace.

Tips: Ask him to lean over to stimulate your clit with his fingertips.

Variations: If it makes things easier and more comfortable, your lover can lean over and be in charge of the thrusting. Consider other types of furniture that allow you to comfortably hang your head for deep throating, e.g., your couch.

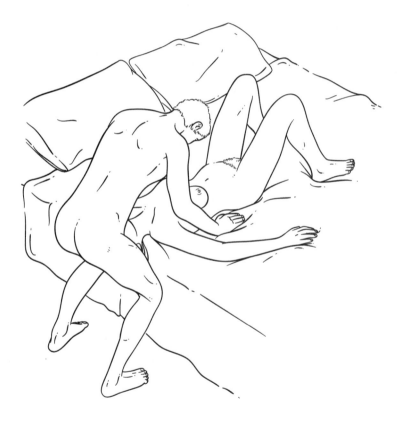

Soixante-Neuf (a.k.a. "69")

Why couples love it: This position holds the ooo-la-la of French sex appeal.

You *and* Him: There are a few ways to work this position so you have some options. You and your lover can either both lie on your sides or take the time to decide who will be on top, facing downward and who will be on the bottom, facing upward. The person on top guides the action.

Tips: Place a pillow under the bottom's head in cases where someone is on top.

Variations:

- Try an almost 69, which is where one partner simply doesn't return the favor.
- Try a 68, where one partner lies down, face up, and the other lies the opposite way, also face up.

Standing 69

Meant for true athletes, standing 69 is more easily done moving from off of 69 on a high-standing bed. In being one of the most challenging variations of soixante-neuf, it needs a bit more attention than the other ones. The "base" partner, who will most likely be your guy, will need to exercise incredible strength in lifting the two of you off of the bed while keeping both of you interlocked in 69. Alternatively, you can approach this version of 69 with one partner assuming headstand while the other stands, supporting their partner's legs. The lover doing the headstand—most likely you—can then slowly be lifted so that mouths and groins meet. In either case, if you're the one upside down it would be helpful to grip the thighs of your standing partner, while strongly squeezing your legs into his sides for support.

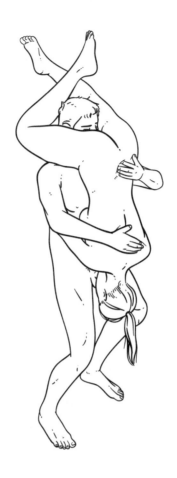

Kneeling or Sitting 69

Depending on your and your lover's heights, you may want to try the kneeling 69, where either you or your lover is on your or his knees. Whether for greater comfort or stability, sitting 69, where the base partner is sitting on the side of a bed or chair, is another variation. Finally, if you have a super-flexible partner, have him bend over all the way as you sit on the floor for a more from-behind angle. You can also spread your legs for variation. Note: If it's hard to have both of you pleasuring at the same time, you or your partner can face the same direction for an advanced version of 68.

| Erotic Furniture and Supports

Pillows, props, bolsters, and other play gear can open your mind to a whole new realm of sexual pleasuring, especially in cases where movement is limited, e.g., during pregnancy, or one person may be hurting. In planning out the ways you want to bend, suspend, prop up, move, or touch your lover, consider the following to add novelty and variety to your oral sex positions:

Sex Swing. This suspension unit's acrylic tubes are placed over the top of your closed door. You then slip your lover's legs into the loops, adjusting them on the thighs. Have your man balance himself with arm handles while you do a little more than lick your lips.

Super Sex Sling. For long-haul oral sex sessions, place this sling's thick pad behind your lover's neck. You can then position him using an adjustable suspension strap, secured with Velcro cuffs.

Positioning Sex Strap. For serious oral sex, the padded strap around the receiving partner's lower waist allows for a comfortable lift.

Sex Furniture. Sold under brand names like Liberator Shapes and Love Pegasus, these soft, but firm padded platforms come in a variety of inclines, platforms, and shapes. Have fun exploring different sexual positions, including those that help to facilitate orgasm and lift your partner's pelvis for better oral sex stimulation.

Sex Savvy

Sex furniture is a must-have for people with disabilities, injuries, or chronic illnesses that make intimacy difficult. In some cases, given one's physical limitation, oral sex, where your lover's legs are placed over your biceps is the only or best kind of sex to be having. Supports can add to one's repertoire.

| Take Your Show on the Road

So, you're ready to realize oral sex in the great outdoors. Whether you're looking at your washing machine, balcony, or shower in a whole new way, or analyzing if oral sex feats involving a closet, car, plane, or train are worth the risk, consider the following matters:

- Mouth access. Just how easy will it be for the lips and genitals to meet?
- Depth. How much of your lover's twig and berries will make it into your mouth?
- Angle. Will the position help to avoid or induce issues like gagging?
- Space. How much do you have to work with?
- Comfort. Will either of you be uncomfortable, especially if you plan to hold your position for a while?

- **Props.** Can the sexual scenario be made comfortable? Are any enhancements needed?
- **Fantasy component.** Other than shaking things up—or running the risk of getting into major trouble in some cases—what can make oral sex outside of the bedroom all that?

Now that you know all of the pretzel poses that make up oral sex coreplay, it's a good idea to get in-the-know to jump start the action—and his reactions. In Chapter 4, we dive into some effective forms of foreplay when it comes to fellatio, whether it's you, him, or his cock that's the appetizer.

Foreplay for Oral Sex

The idea that getting there is half the fun has never been truer than when it comes to seduction. You can't resist your lover's allure, with attempts at the fine art of foreplay often more exciting than the eventual sex act of choice. In bringing the senses to life while stoking the fires of longing, foreplay is a dance between partners that seeks to drive them to the brink of orgasm. With anticipation lending itself to feverish amour, lovers up the ante of pleasures to be had orally in teasing each other to no end with various foreplay scenarios.

Appetizer or Main Course?

Many lovers regard oral sex as a sexy longing to be satiated en route to "bigger and better" things, namely intercourse. With intercourse largely seen as the main course of erotic exchanges between lovers, oral sex is often not given the full attention it deserves. Yet this sensual appetizer can very much be the main event, which allows your and you lover to fully luxuriate in the experience. Instead of being consumed with what's to come, in this book, you can bask between your partner's legs as the star of the show. In fact, approaching oral sex as the main act takes the pressure off, allowing you and your guy more opportunities to bond and be intimate, and more excuses to entice one another. But whether you and your partner are using oral sex as an act of foreplay or the main event, you don't have to head straight downstairs. Take some time and use your mouth for other things before you get down to business.

Sex Q & A

How much foreplay is necessary for having good sex?

Each person's sexual response is determined by a number of physical, psychological, emotional, and relationship factors. A person who is stressed after a hard day at work may require more foreplay in getting in the mood for intimacy, while lovers who have been flirting all day via phone may be ready to get all over each other the moment they meet. In general, mental erotic engagement is more important than anything. It can take mere seconds or many minutes, and is very individual.

Get Back to Basics: Kissing

In our eagerness to pucker up with one's privates, it can be easy to overlook the oral pleasures to be had with the original oral sex—kissing. Physical, emotional, and sexual, a great deal of information is exchanged when our lips meet. The kiss expresses a slew of feelings, like affection, passion, love, need, forgiveness, wanting, and missing. Men in particular use kissing as a way to seduce, and they're quite into puckering up—much more so than they're given credit for.

As a sexual act that is exchanged romantically and/or sexually in over 90 percent of the world's cultures, the kiss is a major mate assessment tool, rated as one of the most romantic acts a couple can partake in. Not surprisingly, kissing is directly proportional to a couple's relationship satisfaction. So no matter where you plan to include oral sex in a sexual session, remember that the original kiss is where you can perfect your technique before going for the genitals.

Sex Savvy

Kissing burns 26 calories per minute. With most people spending 20,160 minutes in a lifetime kissing, that's 524,160 calories burned!

A Kiss Isn't Just a Kiss

Kissing indicates to your lover that you're interested in being sexually intimate to some degree. It can also hint at what you have to offer in the oral department down there; that's part of what makes kissing so exciting, especially in situations where you're not sure just how far exchanges will erotically escalate. Caught up in the moment, you or your lover may be perfectly content playing tonsil hockey and find yourselves doing absolutely nothing more than locking lips. And this is perfectly fine since kissing serves to:

- Promote sexual access sooner or later, with males being particularly clever in using the kiss as a way to lasciviously lure romantic partners.
- Induce bonding and commitment.
- Show your genuine desire and love for one another.
- Invite reconciliation, helping lovers to reunite after a fight.
- Trigger sexual desire with the exchange of testosterone.
- Spike dopamine in the brain, which is associated with romantic love. (The neurotransmitters released with a kiss are the same brain chemicals that go crazy when you sky dive or run a marathon!)
- Cause sexual excitement, which may increase levels of oxytocin in both men and women.

Research out of Lafayette College has found that kissing increases hormones in the brain, setting off a complex chemical process that makes the experience relaxing, exciting, and loving. While women often need extra ambiance, like dim lighting or romantic music, to reach the same state, men have a heightened awareness of these feelings. Researchers aren't sure why this chemical reaction happens, but suspect that it's due to the swapping of hormones in the saliva.

Rolls Off the Tongue

"A great kiss is the ultimate aphrodisiac. If I'm dating someone who is an amazing kisser, I automatically assume that everything else is going to be amazing, including the oral. It's powerful and intoxicating, always leaving me wanting more." } Jaymes

Get Caught Up in Kissing

When it comes to oral endeavors, kissing is a way to mutually teach each other about the techniques you like. It's a way to learn about the rhythms, pressures, and stylistic approaches your lover might enjoy in more place than one. So set out to spend a date simply kissing and nothing else. Focus on the mouth as your prime pleasure center. Your mission: to discover exactly the way your lover wants to be kissed or to experiment with different kissing techniques and styles. Take turns being the lead kisser. When it's his turn to be in charge, ask him to show you what he likes, or simply exhale "Do you like that?" as you come up to breathe from a marathon make-out session. Pay attention, too, to his nonverbal compliments, what he's doing with his body to show you that he's into the action. Erotically escalate the action by responding more enthusiastically with your own kissing. Lick and suck his tongue to plant ideas of what's to come. In taking breathers, lick your way down his treasure trail, stop short of his penis, smile, and work your way back up. Repeat several times.

Sex Savvy

Arrange for a date night that will involve no more than oral coreplay. Such pleasuring makes sex much less goal-oriented, taking the pressure off of lovers to get somewhere, and allowing them to simply enjoy the moment and the sex play at hand.

In giving ample attention to kissing, like with the other oral, be sure to take breathers, gazing into each other's eyes or sprinkling his face, neck, and shoulders with kisses. Keep the moment light with sweet nothings and appreciations. This can act as an incredible tease as to when exactly you may go south, if at all.

For those romantic moments where you really want to get caught up in the kissing (and as a way of not getting too caught up in your head), check in with your bodies every now and then, taking a deep breath as you do so. Encourage him to do the same. This will make your kissing more of a total body experience. During these mini-breaks, share how you're reacting to the situation physically and mentally. Not only does this help both of you to appreciate the moment more, but it helps lovers impart those vital details that can put your other oral endeavors over the top.

Sex Savvy

Get a little crazy with your kissing, trying moves beyond the traditional kiss. This might include tugging your lover's bottom lip with your teeth, or sucking on his tongue when it's in your mouth, or tickling the roof of his mouth with your tongue. With every move, consider how it could be incorporated into your oral efforts.

Lip Care for Better Loving

No matter what kind of kiss you're delivering, you want sexy lips. With a person's face often the first thing that catches another's attention, mouth maintenance becomes critical in evoking positive reactions. Healthy, soft, luscious lips make you look appealing and attractive, a point made even more evident when you think about how having dry, chapped lips can impact one's look negatively. So alluring are the lips that the media can't get enough of featuring Hollywood stars, like Angelina Jolie, who have luscious lips. Looking kissable is irresistible, and it starts with proper lip care.

In making mouth maintenance a regular part of your self-care routine, drink plenty of water and eat a lot of vitamin-rich foods, like fruits and vegetables. Regularly apply lip balm, gloss, or moisturizers year-round, with those containing SPF ideal for maximum sun protection when needed. Lip butter or an aloe lip treatment can also help with moisturizing, keeping your lips soft, soothed, hydrated, and protected. A lip scuff, like that made by the Body Shop, that removes dead skin, can further give you a conditioned feel.

Rolls Off the Tongue

"Supple lips are so inviting, and definitely get me thinking about all of the places I'd like to be kissed—and more." } Kier

Lipsticks for "Kissing Power"

Healthy lips are so important for planting sexy kisses that sex glosses are available in helping lovers last for the long-haul. Make your lips super slick, sexy, plump, and tingly with flavored lip gloss like the Grrl Toyz Slip Sticks Oral Enhancement Sex Gloss. Or play upon the urban legend rainbow parties, giving the illusion that group sex is taking place. Heavily popularized by the media in the early twenty-first century, this urban sex party myth made claim that teen girls would, in sequence, take turns performing oral sex on males, each wearing her own shade of lipstick. Collectively, the girls left a "rainbow" of colors down each guy's shaft. In keeping your lips moist during oral sex, have fun hosting your own rainbow party, realizing that watching you take mini-breaks to reapply a new color can be a sex act in itself.

Sex Q & A

How can I teach my lover what I want done when he goes downtown? I love to give, but I'm hoping he'll return the favor!

Use a direct approach. Simply say, "I'd love it if you tried kissing me (or using your tongue this way) next time you go down on me." Most guys appreciate, and even want, clear direction on what turns you on. If you'd prefer to use a more indirect approach, however, exaggerate the style you desire in your own kissing, even hinting, "I'm so imagining you doing this somewhere else." Your lover will hopefully eventually tune into the rhythm or technique you're trying to establish, realizing that this is what you want. Ask him to do the same if he has trouble telling you want he wants.

| Oral Seductions

Beyond the art of kissing, in working your way to a lover's most titil-lating target zones, you want to build sensations and be a tease. Initiating oral action is your way to take sexiness to a whole new level. Any or a combination of the following seductive strategies are sure to make your partner putty in your hands for other oral attentions in no time.

Look Like You Want Sex

Look cool, calm, and collected, but be ready to pounce when you want to rev things up. This starts with giving your lover longing glances, holding his gaze for a moment and smiling invitingly. Play with your-self; touch places you'd like to be touched later, like your neck. Run your fingers through your hair or play with the buttons on your top. These are all, often unconscious, signals that you're attracted to the guy you're with.

Let Your Lover Know You Want to Perform Oral Sex

Establish a secret signal for those times you want only oral. This might be as simple as drawing an "O" on your lover's lower back to putting on an entire performance. Become the ultimate oral tease by slowly applying lipstick or lip balm in front of your lover, asking him if he has any clue what you're thinking about. You can also tape a flirtatious note to the banana in his lunch bag or send him a sexy email, detailing all of the ways you plan to bring him to climax the next time you're on your knees. Whether your hints are subtle, like sucking on a lollipop, or very direct like whispering "I'm not wearing any underwear," oral efforts are initiated when you get devilishly flirtatious and fresh.

Take Charge

Exuding an attitude of playfulness, confidence, and desire, let your needs be known. This *carpe diem* approach to stimulating desire can be as easy as putting on some music and slow dancing, drawing a sensual bath, playing a romantic movie, or popping in a sex tape that captured your last orgasmic oral endeavor. Remember, your approach sets the tone of the action to come.

Use Your Hands

Warm up your partner's genitals with a nice erotic massage. Bring your lover's erogenous zones to life with some finger action, starting gently at first and slowly building the pace, while gradually applying more pressure. Incorporate some of your favorite lubricant, making things wet in a way that's sexually suggestive.

Seduce with Sound

Stimulate your partner's *auriculogenital reflex* (ear stimulation response) by breathing heavily into his ear. Or practice some sultry sex talk, like "I have to have you," getting as graphic or as dirty as you think your lover will enjoy.

Practice Fresh Breath

It's hard to maintain cool breath when gum isn't the best idea before going down on your lover. You can, however, whip out a fresh breath spritz like Binaca. Tasting like peppermint, spearmint, or cinnamon only makes your mouth all the more inviting.

Slip in a Naughty Movie

Sometimes you need help planting the seed or launching sexual excitement. A steamy flick, X-rated or not, can do just the trick in focusing both you and your lover's minds on more important matters.

Sex Savvy

Keeping things playful is key in maintaining sexual interest in the form of foreplay. Sex toy shops have numerous adult oral sex board games, adding tantalizing tasks to your adventures. They'll have you playing to win as never before, with games like the Oral Sex Board Game. The winner receives oral sex!

Lather Up: Bath and Shower Play

Sometimes all the seduction you need for oral is a little bit of water play. Some lovers like to wash up before oral, mentally cleansing themselves before engaging in this type of sex play. Others like the excuse of getting fresh while freshening up. Even if a shower or bath isn't necessary, it's hard to resist getting naked and running your hands all over your lover's slick body—and where your hands go, it's only natural for your mouth to follow. . . .

Adding to the appeal of water play is that it gives you the perfect excuse to try positions not usually done in bed during oral pursuits, like standing. The warm water also has a relaxing, but invigorating effect, encouraging you and your guy to release the day's tensions and let loose in a most uninhibited way. Finally, the wetness may allow you to bypass the need for lube while still keeping things slick.

Sex Savvy

Take advantage of the showerhead when you and your man experiment with water play. Spray your guy's *glans* while you orally entertain other erogenous zones. Try experimenting with different settings for varying degrees of reactions to see what the two of you like best.

| Role-Playing

When it comes to your erotic imagination, anything can happen—and almost anything can be acted out. Fantasies and sexual storylines can stir the libido, bolster sexual excitement, and add new life to oral "sexplorations." In a relationship defined by trust, good communication, openness, and a sense of adventure, sharing your fantasies during foreplay can be an erotically intense bonding experience. While it can be a bit intimidating and embarrassing to share some of your deepest curiosities, longings, and desires, dishing out sexual imaginings for live passion-filled performances makes for some memorable moments in the bedroom. As you ponder which storylines to share (and not), and which scenarios have the potential for bedroom theater, consider, too, the following orally themed sexual fantasies in launching your riveting role-play efforts.

Rolls Off the Tongue

"Oral sex orgy–style fantasies are some of the hottest I have. Naked, oiled up people all feasting on each other's loins and taking turns on each other . . . it's so taboo and uncommon and racy in being considered so wrong. And it *so* gets me off!" }Magda

- **Virgin Sex.** Pretend you've never given oral sex before and are most eager to be mentored. Be sure to ask for more detailed directions, playing up what you don't know and exaggerating your reactions as to what it's like to lick, taste, and be the perfect pleaser.
- **Stranger Sex.** Plan to meet your lover at a bar, but pretend that you don't know each other. If you're the one hitting on your man, simply say "hello," offer to buy him a drink, make small talk, then ask if he wants to get out of there for a little fun. Don't say a word as you steal off to a secluded location. Your sole focus and concern: giving the best anonymous oral ever.
- **Cop and Careless Driver.** You've just been pulled over for reckless driving. You know you're guilty, but can't afford the ticket and want to avoid jail time. How are you going to get yourself out of the situation? It may simply require offering the nice looking officer some serious oral in the back seat of your car.
- **Psychotherapist and Client.** Normally, you would never think to act inappropriately by taking advantage of a distraught client, but this case is classic Freudian and you have a few ideas on how to best treat your man's arrested development when it comes to oral fixations.

- **Bad Girl Scenario.** You've been a bad girl. The best form of "punishment"? Going down on your guy. Maybe this won't teach you to be a good girl, but, as the saying goes, you'll sure have a lot more fun.
- **Pimp and Whore.** You've already blown your night's earnings and know that your pimp is going to be quite upset that you have no way to pay him his share. Perhaps a nice blow job will suffice for a job well done and an even more generous payout.
- **Dracula Sex.** While your victim's neck is irresistible, there's another erogenous zone you'd rather suck and lick and satiate. In making sure that your victim doesn't get away while being "tortured," tie him up with restraints, like a scarf or handcuffs.

Sex Savvy

Enhance your oral efforts by focusing your lover's attention with a blindfold. Available in soft black microfiber, pleather, leather, silk, and satin, among a host of other fabrics, this tool will force your man to better tune into the sensations, getting more out of the experience.

Exotic Locations

Bold lovers will sometimes take their show on the road, engaging in oral sex in secluded locations or in very public places where action is still quite discreet. In brainstorming all of the places where you might be able to get away with some oral action, consider that getting busted could land you in some legal trouble. Still, with the risk of getting caught a huge part of the erotic thrill, lovers have bragged about where they've been willing to engage in oral, so be cautious, but don't be afraid to take risks.

"My two biggest loves are cars and sex, so I've pursued every kind of road head imaginable—while I'm driving through town, going for a ride in the country, pulled over on the side of an interstate, parked in the pouring rain at a popular look-out-point make-out spot . . . It's always a thrill." } Hank

To keep the thrills coming, consider different ways to eroticize foreplay—based on what you and your guy are really into. Furthermore, be sure to brainstorm all of the different techniques at your disposal that can make for a totally different experience. If you're having trouble getting started, Chapter 5 is chock full of ideas.

Techniques for Oral Sex Aficionados

When it comes to erotic inspiration, new techniques are a way to avoid boredom, revive passion, or make for completely different experiences. With variety-offering novel experiences that keep you and your lover engaged, turned on to oral, and feeling united, changing up the tried and true can be an enjoyable conquest. Even if you don't have much experience giving head, employing different tactics during your trial-and-error period can help you discover what your guy is into and what turns him on. No matter the situation, trying out new techniques for oral sex adds spice and never-before-known sensations, upping your aptitude for impressing any lover.

Oral Sex Basics

When it comes to giving good head, a number of techniques can be used to awaken, accelerate, and amplify arousal in stimulating your guy's genitals with your mouth. Major moves include licking, lapping, flicking, slurping, circling, tickling, sucking, kissing, pressing, and nibbling a particular hot spot or his entire penis. The pace can range anywhere from fast to slow, with pressure anywhere from hard to soft. Patterns of movements across erogenous zones can be side to side, up and down, diagonal, or circles. Pick up any popular press magazine and they're likely daring you to skillfully try drawing the alphabet or figure eights with the tip of your tongue to get the blood down there flowing even more.

The key in figuring out what your guy enjoys is to add a little variety from one sex session to the next. Changing up the technique also helps to prolong sexual intimacy; if you don't want him to come right away you want to switch things up. For example, you can experiment with different parts of your mouth to create different sensations, like repeatedly rubbing the really soft inside of your lips across one of his erogenous zones. Using various parts of the tongue can also make for an entirely different experience, especially given that you can make it soft, pointed, firm, etc.

No matter what you choose to do, start out slowly, building up the rhythm. Keep in mind that maintaining consistency when it comes to pressure and pace is what brings a lover to orgasm. This is what men like more than anything. This is what they do to themselves manually when they masturbate. If you do otherwise you'll throw him for a loop, disrupting his concentration and ability to get into the sensations. However, making, then breaking, contact from time to time can help to build sexual tension when done skillfully.

More than anything though, as you work to make him putty in your hands, maintain your enthusiasm. Acting like you're into it—even if you're not—means more to him than anything else going on.

Rolls Off the Tongue

"Enthusiasm. All of these questions boil down to enthusiasm. If you're going to go down there, make me believe that you are having the time of your life. That is what will give *me* the time of *my* life!" } Tyron

Part of your enthusiasm when going down may be related to your confidence level. Don't let any doubts hold you back. Fake it until you can make it happen for real. You're not hurting anybody by acting like you know what you're doing. You're only making the experience better for him by taking your time, keeping your cool, and feeling good about yourself and what's going on.

Sex Q & A

How do you put on a condom using only your mouth?

Carefully put a nonlubricated condom in your mouth, reservoir tip pointing towards your throat and the ring of the condom in front of your teeth. Use your tongue to press the tip against the roof of your mouth since this keeps air out of the rubber. (If your partner desires lube for greater sensitivity, then have him squirt some in at this point.) Place one or both of your hands at the base of your lover's penis. Press the tip of the condom against the head of the penis. (If your partner is uncircumcised, pull back his foreskin before lowering your head to put the condom on.) Roll the condom down his penis using your lips, carefully avoiding the use of your teeth.

Warming Up His Groin

When going down on a guy, you can use your oral talents to make him erect—he'll often get hard quickly. Or you can use your hands or other means of foreplay, like a seductive strip tease or playing with yourself to get him hard before you take his penis into your mouth. Send shivers down his spine by dragging your fingers up and down his inner thighs, selectively planting kisses to the area around his groin, and teasing him by being so close, but still so far away. To get him hotter, give his cock nice, long licks, as though thoroughly enjoying an ice cream cone. Alternatively, you can employ your oral talents while he's still in his boxers. Simply wet the fabric with your tongue, bringing his cock to life, if it isn't already, by puffing quick blasts of hot air onto it. (Just take care not to do this at the tip.)

Sex Q & A

What are some moves to incorporate during rimming?

When eating your man out during analingus, you may want to suck or circle the area of the anal opening. You can also "dip" your tongue into the opening. At the end of the day, you can basically use a lot of the same mouth, lip, and tongue moves that you use during other types or oral stimulation, depending on your lover's preferences. You may, though, have to spend more time stroking your partner's penis in keeping your lover relaxed, as the vulnerability factor of rimming may make him more uptight during this type of oral action.

Despite meaning "to suck," *fellatio* involves a whole lot more. Whether you're getting him warmed up or dazzling him with tantalizing tactics throughout an oral sex session, you can impress him by licking his entire shaft from base to tip, covering every bit with your saliva.

After you've wet the entire area, blow cool air onto it to make his hair stand on end. Occasionally, swirl your tongue around the head as a tease, before finally resting it flat on the glans or foreskin. If your lover is uncircumcised, push back his foreskin to lick his glans or sweep your tongue under it.

Alternatively, you can lick the urethral opening or stimulate it using a flicking motion. Be sure to check in with him as you do this since this will not turn on some guys; he may want your abilities focused elsewhere.

| Attending to the Penis

Before taking your lover into your mouth, be sure to cover your teeth with your lips, creating a loose, soft "O" shape with your mouth. Take his entire cock into your mouth and have it rest there for a couple of seconds. Now have it glide slowly out. Pause dramatically, then repeat a couple of times, choosing to lick the frenulum underneath the tip with either your tongue's tip or the flat part of your tongue.

Sex Savvy

Don't let hair be an issue. Ask your guy to help you hold your long locks if they're getting in the way. If your partner's pubic hairs are an issue, lick from the inside out which allows them to stick together in a matted down fashion.

Now mimic thrusting by moving his member in and out of your mouth as you slowly tighten your lips around his shaft and use your tongue to apply additional pressure. The tongue action can be circular, quick, or lingering, or involve more of a licking or pressing up against his penis's hot spots. Or experiment with different types of tongue movements—swirls, darting, massaging—providing different kinds of stimulation until you know you've struck gold. No matter what you choose, remember to always check in with him that it feels good. (Note: Grunts and head nod responses are perfectly acceptable.)

Covering as much surface area as possible, push your lover's erect penis up toward his stomach while licking the underside of his shaft. Keep your tongue flat as you move your head from side to side. Then strategize your next move. Will it be giving his glans a nice counter-clockwise massage? Flicking your tongue across his corona? Rocking your lips across his frenulum? No matter what, take your time, building the action and your momentum. Unless the situation requires it, most men are in no rush and love the build-up.

Continue to play away, only more rapidly. Loosen your throat muscles and take him deeper, breathing through your nose to avoid gagging. For added sensation, move your hand up and down the shaft, as though milking it, in rhythm with the penile thrusting of your mouth, getting faster and faster, or incorporate any of the suggestions outlined in the next section.

Sex Savvy

While sucking brings more blood to an erogenous zone, too much sucking action can be uncomfortable, so avoid going overboard.

| Make Use of Your Hands

When going down on your guy, try stimulating him in more ways than one. Keep one hand gripped at the base of his shaft, as this will help you to maintain control of his movements and have the other "chase" your mouth as it slides up and down his shaft. Generate as much saliva as you can for a natural hand lube, keeping things wet and comfortable. In the early going, when you reach the head of your lover's penis, pull your mouth away to let your chaser hand slip around the head for a nice grip before sliding back down the shaft. For variety, twist your hand as you slide it up and down, or just twist it at the tip. Doing a quick hand twist as your head bobs up and down his shaft can also accelerate things. As you tease the tip of your man's penis with the tip of your tongue, take his shaft between your hands and rub it as though trying to start a fire, or press against the sides of his shaft, as though praying for a more heavenly hand stroke. You can also form a ring with your thumb and index finger around the base of the shaft, and use this as a moving cock ring.

To intensify his orgasm, massage his perineum in a circular motion by pressing two of your fingers into the area about one inch behind his balls (you'll feel this as a dent) about thirty seconds before you sense that he's going to cum. As he orgasms, squeeze the base of his penis. Invite him to shoot his load all over your chest or to give you the prized pearl necklace, if you'd like.

Sex Savvy

Unless your lover is into it, avoid giving hickies or using your teeth, especially to the point of leaving bite marks. Ask if your lover finds either of these forms of stimulation a turn-on before leaving him black and blue!

| Play with His Sac

Try not to leave your lover's balls out of the picture. Lick them lightly before taking one or both into your mouth for some gentle sucking known as *teabagging*. Enhance the experience by twirling your tongue or massaging the testicle gently as though trying to get peanut butter off of the roof of your mouth. Or try licking the skin between his balls before giving each your undivided attention.

You can also try lifting up his sac and flicking your tongue across the crease of skin where his scrotum meets the body. And, if your mouth is elsewhere, keep the scrotal sac charged by cupping it or dragging your nails up the inside of his thighs and over his scrotum. Pulling the sac as he's about to orgasm can make for an even more intense experience.

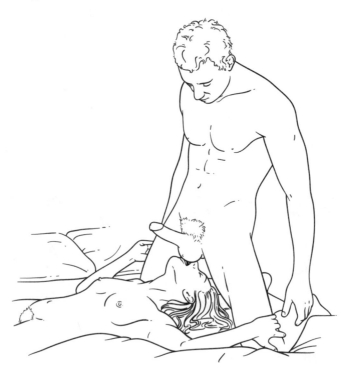

Tongue Kung Fu

Tongue Kung Fu is an ancient Chinese approach to skillfully and consciously giving or receiving oral sex. It's where you skillfully combine the use of your tongue, teeth, lips, and intention in providing pleasure to bolster feelings of connectedness and passion. The following are some of the major techniques:

- Tongue diving. Use the full length and strength of your tongue to directly "dive" into your lover's groin. Such an act is seen in this ancient Chinese art as expressing your heart, since the tongue is seen as an extension of the heart.
- Tongue flutters. Rapidly flutter your tongue back and forth across your lover's hot spots, as though this muscle is a vibrator.
- Tongue scooping. Form your tongue in a spoon shape to use in a come-hither motion on a hot spot, like his perineum.

Sex Savvy

Avoid touching your lover's glans after he has climaxed. His erogenous zones are going to be super sensitive post-sex play, and will need a bit of a breather before they're handled again.

Oral Sex Made Easier

No matter your plan, issues may come up that have the potential to throw off your game. Be open to and ready for anything. Tune into your lover's sounds and bodily reactions to gauge if things are going well. Ask, if it's not obvious, if your partner is thoroughly enjoying himself. Finally, don't be afraid to incorporate maneuvers and sex tips that come to you on the spot, like licking in rhythm to music that's playing, or humming to become your own vibrating sex toy, or twisting your tongue in ways that only your genes allow. Who knows what could end up feeling good? Approach your oral sex efforts with the idea that the sky is the limit.

Sex Savvy

If your partner has a piercing, be careful with your teeth. If possible, flip the jewelry out of the way. Otherwise, consider how the piercing can add to the stimulation factor.

Afterplay

You're basking in the glow of some out-of-this-world oral sex, but don't let things end there! Just as with other types of sex, afterplay is an important way to top off a satisfying experience, helping the feelings and sensations last. So instead of falling asleep or making for the door, kiss and hold each other afterward. Take a bath or shower together while on your sex high. Talk about how nice the sex was, especially if your partner is trying to get over issues with oral. Allow yourselves the chance to recharge, because you never know when you just have the room to have a little bit more.

Rolls Off the Tongue

"Coming down from oral sex is one of the most magical parts of it. It's like you're in your own world and you have all of these feel-good chemicals coursing through your body. Lingering helps them to stay a little longer." } Charlotte

As with any good performance, a few rehearsals may be necessary. Your show can also call for a standing ovation with just the right props. Chapter 6 arms you with some of the most effective sexual enhancements for your—and his—pleasure.

It's Playtime! Sensual Enhancements

What's in your treasure chest? After reading this chapter, you may just have to add to whatever you already own, as the occasional investment in erotic enhancements can do wonders for your sex life. Treating yourselves to practically anything of the "for adults only" assortment can introduce new sensations, variety, and lust-filled experiences when it comes to your oral efforts. With the sexual and sensual accoutrements numbering into the thousands, sorting through what's best for your passionate pleasuring can feel overwhelming. Here, we seek to make your next online or in-store shopping experience all the easier, by highlighting the most tempting goodies when it comes to oral sex enhancement.

Lubricants

You want his cock even wetter when you're going down and he's definitely with you on that one. Why? Because a wet mouth is reminiscent of a wet vagina—every guy's goal. But which lube to use is a common question from lovers since there are so many types of lubricants on the market. Making matters even more confusing is knowing which ones are best for oral sex. Ample amounts of lube can enhance your oral experiences, so, without further ado, here are your choices:

Flavored lubricants. Found at drugstores, adult shops (both online and physical), and other retail stores with sexual health products, flavored lubes were originally developed to help mask the smell and taste of condoms, primarily during oral sex. Latex safe, they can be used with sex toys as well. Depending on your preferred brand and flavor, the scent and taste can enliven the senses, making oral sex a more appetizing event. Oral sex becomes a delectable experience when made more scrumptious with sensual seasonings of sorts, like mojito peppermint, pomegranate vanilla, and chocolate orange blends offered by sex toy companies like Babeland.

Flavored lubes do, however, have their drawbacks, in that they can:

- Dry quickly (though with saliva or water, they can become slick again).

- Stain sheets or be hard to wash out if they're a certain color.
- Be too sticky for other forms of sex, like self-pleasuring.

Be sure to test the products before use, testing for allergies by dabbing a spot on an area of both your inner arm and his; to check for a potential reaction. If you're good to go, have a ball trying different ones to see which ones you and your partner like best.

Water-based lubricants. Though they tend to dry faster than other types of lubes, water-based lubricants tend to be the most user-friendly, i.e., nonirritating, and easy to clean, overall.

Silicone lubes. While these can be used, ingesting too much can lead to upset stomach. If you want to do silicone, make sure it's a high-quality one, as in free of cyclopentasiloxane, which can sometimes taste a bit like petroleum.

Oil-based lubricants: These should not be used if you're practicing safe sex, since these can compromise the latex. And even if you're not using a condom or dental dam, applying an oil-based lube for oral action can be gross. Use at your own risk.

Warming lubricants. Available in flavors like hot buttered rum and blueberry, these lubes heat up when you rub them onto your lover's body. Blow on the area to heat things up even more. Just be sure to test an area of your partner's skin first, as some people do not like the sensations these lubes provide.

| Edible Aphrodisiacs

After a more savory seductive experience? Aphrodisiacs are any food, drink, drug, smell, or item believed to attract or invite sexual desire, or increase your level of sexual excitement. So an aphrodisiac can basically be anything you or your guy find stimulating, giving you a great deal of power over what edibles to introduce to oral efforts. Plus, experimenting with different edibles only adds to the adventure, helping you and your lover bond. In deciding on the aphrodisiac of your choice, you may want to consider some of the most popular of all time for upping your oral efforts:

- Champagne. Drizzle some sparkling wine on your partner's abdomen, and have fun chasing the streams of bubbly—in their many directions—with the tip of your tongue.
- Cinnamon. Sprinkle some of this aromatic spice on his prized possession before licking him absolutely clean.
- Fruit. Between their sexy shapes, textures, and juices, you can have a field day with fruits in suggesting where you want to take the action or making things a bit tastier. Rub sticky juices from fruit like papaya, peach, orange, and mango on your lover's groin—and then lick it all off.
- Chocolate. Acclaimed throughout the ages for its supposed sexual effects, this sweet will make you and your lover happier thanks to its key ingredients: caffeine, anandamide and phenylethylamine or PEA (a natural antidepressant), and theobromine, which boosts endorphin production for a body high. Heat edible dark, white, and milk chocolates, available as novelty body paints, and apply all over your guy's body as tasty foreplay before you get down to business. Alternatively, you can melt chocolate body fondue and paint it all over yourself for sweet seduction. Smear body icing or pour chocolate syrup down your lover's treasure trail for an even tastier treat. In any case, consider going for dark chocolate, since it's known to be a vasodilator, increasing blood flow throughout the body, including the genitals.
- Honey. Dribble this sweet on your lover's most intimate bits for a natural sugar high. Want to avoid the sticky mess? Pull a candy

cock ring around his shaft for double the dessert. Or spray some whipped cream along his groin and nipples or anywhere else you want to feed on your delicacy.

Accessories for Oral Pleasuring

In addition to edibles, there are a whole host of sex toys designed specifically for oral pleasuring in addition to your lips and tongue. Have a blast adding to the sensations or taking them to an entirely new level with some of the following:

Tongue vibe. Slip this vibrating tongue ring onto your tongue for tingly action. Available in glow-in-the-dark, this vibe has a powerful two-speed setting. Screaming O sells a waterproof, disposable version of the tongue vibrator, called the LingO, which is held in place with a stretchy band. The long-lasting motor is ideal for if your tongue ever gets tired.

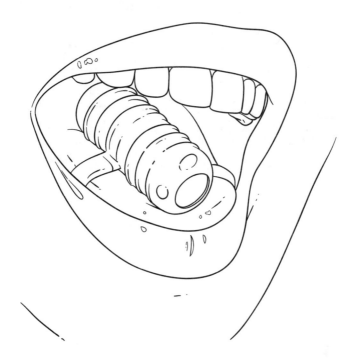

Sqweel. Double the oral action. Packed with ten soft, velvety tongues, this rotating wheel simulates oral sex when you roll it across your lover's hot spots with your hand. NOTE: This battery-powered toy doesn't vibrate, but the wheel rotates to one of three speed options.

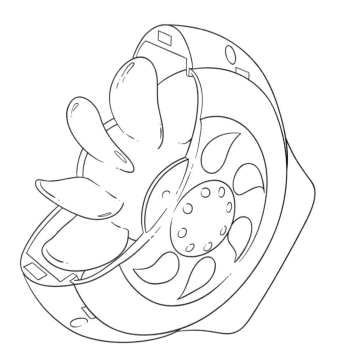

Vibrators. We think of vibrators as being just for women, but they can be used to pleasure your guy's hot spots too. Tease his member by using any kind of powerful vibe against your cheek, when going down on him, so that the vibrations in your mouth make their way to his cock.

Dildo. Fulfill your third-party fantasy by slipping this toy into your partner's nether crevices for full penetration, without the vibration, during oral sex.

Butt plug. Available in different sizes and shapes (ribbed, smooth, or bumpy), slowly insert this toy into your partner's anus for more fullness during tongue action. Alternatively, you can thrust the butt plug in and out of his rectum as you home in on his frenulum or corona. Note: Make sure the butt plug has a flared base so that it doesn't accidentally

slip inside. Don't be surprised, too, if it
shoots out as he reaches climax.

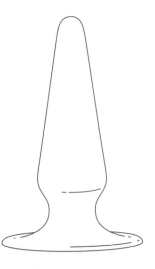

Anal beads. To intensify your lover's
orgasm, have anal beads in place, ready to
stimulate the nerve endings of his anus,
while giving him a nice prostate massage.
These typically five plastic or latex beads
are strung together on a nylon or cotton cord. You want to insert each into his
rectum, using lots of lube, one at a time
while stimulating his cock. As he starts to
approach climax, slowly and gently pull at
the anal beads using the ring at the end.

Sex Savvy

Keep anal beads clean by putting a condom over them and
knotting the end of the condom. You can also stick with nylon
strings and latex beads since these are best when it comes
to cleanliness and disinfecting. Oh, and it practically goes
without saying, but never substitute any random objects, like
his golf balls, when it comes to this kind of sex play.

Cock rings. Stretch one of these love rings over his shaft (or a dong)
for extra sensation. A vibrating cock ring can further blow him away as
you firmly slide your hand up and down his shaft, the tip of your tongue
meeting the tip of his cock for a little massage.

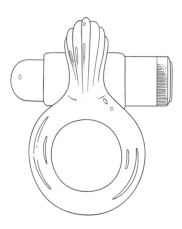

Cock Sleeve. Also called a male stimulator, this toy has two open ends, so you can slide it down your lover's well-lubricated shaft to the base. Push the top of the product down so that the head of his penis sticks out. Now work your magic, focusing all of your attention on the glans and foreskin. This is really great for situations where you don't want to deep throat; the stimulator acts as a buffer for you while still providing stimulation to the rest of his shaft.

Rolls Off the Tongue

"We use sex toys on occasion for variety, especially for those times when you're in the mood, but don't want to do all of the work. The toys are a good excuse for those times we want to pleasure, but are feeling a bit lazy. Nobody is insulted. Both of us are happy." } Bobby

Some other goodies that can spice up your sex life include the following:

Massage mitt. Found at spas, sex toy shops, or your local drugstore, these love gloves come in different textures, like fur and studs, for true magic hands.

Sport sheet. Going to bed never sounded as good as it does with these bondage sheets. Used as regular bed sheets, they typically come with four Velcro restraints, one at each corner, for some serious "have you been a bad boy?" sexperiences.

DVDs. Buy a DVD on oral sex (check out recommendations in the Resources section), where you'll visually learn how to assume oral sex positions, topped off with tips on technique. Not in the mood for instruction? Rent an X-rated film that's all about oral, or find an amateur download online. Either way, you have thousands to choose from!

While there's always caution (and common sense) to be used in experimenting with items found around the house, look at the items you already have in your space. You may not necessarily have to shop at a sex toy store when you have things like a:

- **Mirror.** View your XXX-efforts in a whole new light. Caution: Seeing you work away from all angles will detonate him in no time!
- **Nylon stocking.** Gently wrap this fabric around the base of his penis, then have it chase your lips up and down his shaft, for added sensations. Some men do have a nylon fetish, and for good reason.
- **Camcorder.** Instead of worrying about capturing the moment, have your camcorder rolling so your lover can appreciate the action all over again later on.

Rolls Off the Tongue

"My girlfriend and I admittedly try some of those oral sex tips you read about in magazines like *Cosmo*. Sometimes they do nothing for us. Other times, it's like *wow*! Give me more of that!" }Paul

When it comes to sexual enhancements, your biggest concern is safety first in evaluating its pleasure potential. The sexual situation, like the sacred sex covered in the following chapter, can also determine what toys feel appropriate for the mood you're trying to create. That said, the sky is the limit in what goodies can be a part of your sex play. So see the universe—and everything in it—as the turn on that it is!

CHAPTER 7

Sacred Oral Sex Approaches

It's time to take an "om" moment. After all, raw, unbridled sex can present itself in more ways than one, and ancient Eastern approaches to sex certainly have a worldwide reputation for taking you—and your lover—to bliss and back. Stripping down to the core can make for some of your most unrestrained sexual pursuits and exhilarations, with sacred sex perhaps being the best vehicle for unleashing such.

Sacred sex is an approach to lovemaking that seeks to join and celebrate your and your lover's bodies, minds, and souls. This spiritual discipline taps your sexual energy, which is seen as an embodiment of divine energy. This energy can be intensified and carried through the body via the breath, and other practices, setting every nerve ablaze. Sex is seen as a vehicle for enlightenment, a way to attain an altered state of cosmic unity.

The Allure of Sacred Sex

Realizing transcendence and oneness with your partner, nature, and a higher spirit is done over an extended period of time, with you and your lover riding a roller coaster of sexual response. It is during peak sexual activity, including extended orgasms, that you are launched into cosmic unity. While such can be experienced occasionally and spontaneously, it is with practice that lovers can consciously invite spiritual sexual union. This involves a tuning into your senses, harnessing your sensual and sexual energy, and living fully and presently in every moment.

Sacred sex has been practiced for over 5,000 years, stemming from Hindu and Buddhist practices in India and Tibet. Best known in the form of Tantric sex, sacred sex is based on the belief system that a fusion of sexual energies is the union of each lover's masculine and feminine principles (yin and yang). Joining these opposite forces through lovemaking is seen as a way to achieving union with the Divine.

Sacred sex continually attracts lovers worldwide by not only promising personal and spiritual growth, but for holding the key to a more passionate sex life as well. Couples who practice sacred sex feel greater emotional balance, enhanced self-worth, and greater energy. The quality of their relationship improves, made only sweeter with ecstatic sexual experiences, longer sex sessions, and more powerful sexual reactions.

"We decided to take a sacred sex workshop more for kicks than anything. But once we got into the practice, we were sold. It's no joke. Sacred sex has enhanced every aspect of lovemaking for us. With oral sex in particular, it feels more like a partner worship experience, with an emphasis on undying adoration and love." } Julian

Oral Sex and the *Kama Sutra*

Written around A.D. 350, the *Kama Sutra* is the original, classic guide to extraordinary lovemaking. Written by the Indian philosopher Vatsyayana, this work was penned in an effort to help prevent divorce via good sex. After all, happy couples make for happy marriages. With oral sex in particular, Vatsyayana held that all sexual loving starts with kisses. This oral fixation is what sparks passion, sexual excitement, and the desire for more body touch. Lovers are to then work their way down from a partner's face, lips, throat, and chest to the arms, legs, and "joints of the thighs." The *Kama Sutra* encourages lovers to explore different kinds of kisses and ways each can arouse, with the nurturance of each kiss recognized as very pleasurable and reassuring.

An entire chapter of the *Kama Sutra* focuses on *auparishtaka*, or "oral congress." *Oral congress* involves eight highly descriptive ways of performing fellatio. For our purposes, focus is given to what the *Kama Sutra* has to offer to help you please your partner, as well as other tricks of the trade practiced by Tantric practitioners.

Planning Your Seductions

Set the stage for sacred oral sex by creating a sensual environment. Influence the ambiance of your love chamber with happy pictures of you and your lover, candles, bells, fruit, bowls, shells, plush pillows, oriental rugs, and tapestries. When creating a sacred space, set up an altar in your bedroom or a special spot of your home that is only accessed by you and your lover. Decorate this members-only area with offerings, special items like candles, fresh flowers, and poetry. Include objects that represent your *yoni* (vulva), like almonds, fresh apricots, or triangles, as well as items that represent your guy's *lingam* (penis), like crystals and wands. Add a final touch to your altar offering, by placing a light stone on a dark velvet cushion or a dark stone on a light cushion. Stones to consider for their symbolism are the diamond for everlasting love; the ruby for a very deep, passionate love affair; pearls for long-lasting love; red jasper for warm, sensuous love; or the garnet for sexual pleasure.

Finally, consider how your use of color, lighting, fabrics, and scents in the bedroom are (or aren't) creating a warm, harmonious, peaceful, and comfortable space. Hanging a violet silk, chiffon, or muslin fabric can invite female sexual energy, if so desired, while going for more red will stimulate his vitality and life force.

| *Lingam* Kisses

The *Kama Sutra*'s oral congress techniques range from tender and loving to intense and climax-inducing. Whether you've set the stage for sacred sex or are hoping to add more flair to your fellatio delivery, the following can be approached in sequence or mixed up. You pick and choose the way you want to handle his *lingam* with any of the following:

Nimita ("The Nominal Congress")

Begin this simple, mild technique by holding your lover's *lingam* in your hands and placing the tip lightly between your lips. Move your head in tiny circles. Slowly move the *lingam* around in your mouth, pressing the shaft with your lips, and letting the tongue dance around the head of the penis, before releasing it and softly pulling away your mouth.

Parshvatoddashta ("Biting the Sides")

For this technique, cover the head of his *lingam* with your fingers, which are formed together in a flower bud shape. Now press the sides of the *lingam* with your lips and teeth. Give each side individual attention, alternating firm and soft pressure as you caress the length of the shaft with your mouth.

Bahiha-samdansha ("Pressing Outside" or "Outer Pincers")

Press the end of your lover's *lingam* with your lips, which are closed together. With these pursed lips, kiss it tenderly using a gentle sucking motion, pulling at its soft skin as if you're drawing it out. Put the *lingam* farther into your mouth and press it with your lips. Then take it out, kissing the end.

Antaha ("Inside Pressing" or "Inner Pincers")

Put the *lingam* further into your mouth and press it firmly with your lips before sucking on it. Take it out of your mouth, then repeat as desired.

Rolls Off the Tongue

"I always know I'm in for one of these special techniques because my sweetie puts a lot more time into setting the stage and making sure that I'm comfortable. The extra pampering is a nice added touch and everything makes what she's doing not your average blow job." } Russ

Chumbitaka ("Kissing")

Hold your lover's *lingam* in your hand and kiss it fiercely along its entire length, using your lower lip in a sucking motion.

Parimrshtaka ("Rubbing")

Touch his *lingam* with your tongue everywhere using a flicking motion, then pass your tongue over the end of it with a striking motion, tongue pointed.

Amrachushita ("Sucking the Mango")

Put half of your man's *lingam* in your mouth, then forcibly kiss and vigorously suck on it, as though stripping a mango clean.

Sangara ("Swallowing Up")

Typically done near climax, put the entire *lingam* into your mouth and take it to the very back of your throat. Work your lips and tongue on the shaft until your lover reaches climax.

Sex Savvy

Anoint one another. Honor your lover's body as a temple of your spirit by offering the body as a gift to the Other and the universe. Mix an essential oil, like rose, with an oil base, like pure vegetable oil. Then anoint each other's hearts with dabs of this concoction. Alternatively, you can mix sandalwood essential oil with an oil base and apply drops of this mixture to the area between your lover's eyebrows to awaken his Third Eye, the area between your eyebrows representing your sixth chakra (energy center).

The Crow, a.k.a. "69"

Referred to as *the crow*, *Kakila*, or *congress of crow*, the 69 position takes on great symbolism in the *Kama Sutra*. The Crow is seen as having great mystical powers, including the ability to dissolve substances, transforming original states into fusion form. In assuming 69, lovers are said to be "pecking" at each other's tender love parts like pecking crows, nibbling here and there, pleasing, and making delightful sounds like crows sometimes do. This kissing of the lower parts can employ any of the techniques mentioned in this chapter for sensation and pleasure.

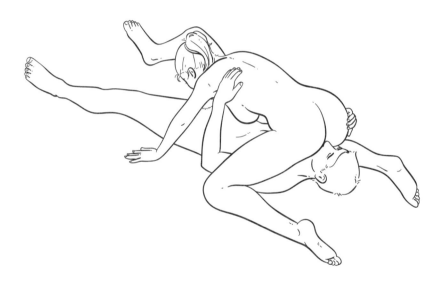

For some couples, sacred sex may be the way to go, at least initially, in developing comfort as a giver or receiver of oral sex. There are a number of issues that can impact you or your partner's ability to let go and fully enjoy the moment. If a sacred sex approach doesn't do the trick, hopefully the tips given in the next chapter on oral sex hang-ups will help to nip issues in the bud once and for all.

CHAPTER 8

Owning Your Pleasures: Assessing Any Issues

By now, you've gone from oral sex amateur to authority. Still, you may find yourself needing to perfect your pleasuring pursuits because it feels as though there's something wanting. In other cases, you—or your partner—may be fielding some issues that are trumping your game. This chapter is all about making sure that the two of you steer clear of anything that can throw your erotic efforts off course!

| Common Mistakes People Make

Whether new to any type of sex or new to a partner, people will often need a few test runs before figuring out the right formula for flawless frolicking. Knowing which blunders to avoid ahead of time can have you presenting yourself as his best blow job queen ever right from the start. Here are the more common ways givers foil their own efforts:

You Don't Recognize the Need for Diversity

While there are generalities that can be made about human sexuality, the truth of the matter is that we're all very individual in our preferences, desires, wants, needs, and responses. Every one of us is unique, sexually speaking, so realize that what might have worked for your last guy isn't going to necessarily work for this one. You have to approach a new partner as a clean slate, testing different moves and discovering what works (and doesn't) when it comes to upmost pleasuring. You also have to put aside any ego issues in the feedback he gives you as well. He's hopefully telling you what he likes and needs without sounding critical. Him being able to share in such a way should be seen as a compliment in that he can be open with you and not an indicator of something you're doing wrong.

Even after you figure out the right formula, you'll want to change up oral on occasion. Nothing spells sexual disaster like same old, same old. So consider novel ways to spice things up in keeping both of you interested in the oral action. Diversity is key.

Your Fangs Get in on the Feast

While a man's penis can handle a lot more than it's usually given credit for, most men are not into teeth. So, unless he's into the occasional scrape, nick, or bite, avoid letting your canines get in on the action. You can solve this problem by wrapping your lips around your teeth when you go down on your man.

You Ignore His Other Hot Spots

It's easy to get lost in the focus of your attention, but your lover's body is covered with erogenous zones that are just dying for some equal attention. So don't ignore your lover's nipples, balls, perineum, back of the knees, etc., just to name a few of the favorite parts within arm's reach.

You Manhandle His Scrotum

It is super fun to play with a guy's balls, but any yanking, hard pulling, grabbing, and squeezing will generally leave them—and him—feeling like they're getting kicked around. While you're striving to be the best, this isn't the World Cup. For most men, this area needs to be handled delicately. So gently tug, rub, or lick them, and check in with him to find out what feels good and just how much more of the same he desires.

You're Not Present

You had a tough day at work; you're feeling blimpy and unsexy from gorging yourself at dinner; you're wondering when you'll find the time tomorrow to pick up your dry cleaning. . . . There could be a million reasons why you're not into oral. But even if you're not into the moment, pretend that you are. Make sure that your hands are busy, exaggerate your head movements, make some noise, and pretty soon you may even start to believe your own performance and really get into everything you're doing.

You Give Up Control

He's getting the blow job of his life and wants more. While a pat on the back should involve a nice pat on the head, it definitely should *not* involve grabbing your head and upping the thrusting action. If he wants it harder or faster, he needs to ask you if you can provide him with more vigorous stimulation, or if you can become even more robust in what you're doing. Otherwise, you could not only potentially resent how he got carried away, but get hurt. No joke.

According to a 1980 article in *Military Medicine,* a teen patient had a black and blue blotch in the back of her throat. Her dentist had to ask her father to leave the room before inquiring if she had a boyfriend. As suspected, the oral sex she was performing on him helped to explain why the mass of tissue near her tonsils was so bruised. The only way to avoid situations like these is to make sure he knows how to ask nicely.

Rolls Off the Tongue

"I had a lover back in college who used to always grab my head to steer the action when I was giving him head. That, and the fact that he was an asshole, still leaves a bad taste in my mouth (pun intended) when I think about how disrespectful and awful it was. Needless to say, I didn't go down on him very often, and will never tolerate such treatment from somebody again." }Christiana

| The Need to Breathe

Drowning yourself in someone else's pleasure can be intoxicating. But it's anything but erotic when you have trouble surfacing for a little air. If you find yourself needing to catch your breath, some quick remedies to the situation include:

- Tilt your head slightly to the side to breathe through one nostril.
- Breathe through your nose, an effort made easier in staying above the sheets.
- Use your fingers to keep the action going when you come up for a breather.

In addition, there are some more advanced tactics that you can employ to keep your passageways open for easier air supply.

Circular Breathing

Circular breathing is an ancient technique that enables an instrumentalist (clarinet, oboe, saxophone, skin flute, etc.) to maintain airflow (and thus sound) through an instrument for a long period of time via inhalation through the nose. Basically, this technique allows you to inhale while you're exhaling, with the "exhale" based on your ability to fill the cheeks with air when you start to run low on the oxygen in your lungs and force it out as you inhale. It involves four stages:

1. As you become low on air, your cheeks puff.
2. Air from your cheeks is pushed through the instrument. Your cheek muscles allow you to maintain the sound while you breathe through your nose.
3. As the air in the cheeks decreases, and sufficient air is inhaled into the lungs through your nose, the soft palate in your throat closes and the air in your lungs is exhaled.
4. Your cheeks resume their normal position.

It is the switching back and forth from the air in the lungs to the air in the cheeks that enables a person to master circular breathing. Know that this doesn't come easily and does require practice. In mastering this effort, it is best to consult books and online resources, written by music instructors, offering circular breathing exercises. Need incentive? The world record for circular breathing runs at almost ninety minutes of continuous playing of a wind instrument. Think about what that can do for your oral efforts.

Yawn

Open your throat muscles with a good yawn. Singers will often overcome throat tightness, especially in reaching high notes, by relaxing their strained throat muscles. So go ahead and yawn loudly. This not only allows your breathing to pass through without obstruction, it awakens you. Just be sure to explain to your lover what you're doing, lest you come off as being rude and bored!

| Common Concerns for You

Oral sex should be a stimulating, gratifying, amazing experience for both you and your guy alike. But there are times when concerns can get in the way of your ability to fully embrace oral eroticism. Here are just some of the issues that could be trumping you or your lover's game . . .

Self-Perceptions

Am I doing this right? Am I good enough? Do I look ridiculous? How long until we reach orgasm? These are just some of the thoughts that can course through your mind as you're going down on somebody. If you find yourself caught up in such worries, stop and focus on the action, and make a mental note to talk to your lover later to make sure that none of your concerns are actual issues. You may just need some serious private reflection time where you confront the way you harshly judge yourself. Ask yourself how your line of thinking could be contributing to your sense of inadequacy.

Guilt Blocks

Sadly enough, some lovers do not feel worthy of receiving affection. For whatever past reasons, they've been made to feel that their sexual feelings, thoughts, and actions are wrong. Ultimately, their sense of well-being when intimate is compromised and they are helpless to make the changes needed to overcome being their own worst enemies. If this is your story consider consulting with a sex counselor or therapist in figuring out how to get to a better place and address what's needed from within, from your relationship, or from your partner to help you accept the joys of oral sex.

Gagging

Hands down one of the biggest concerns—and deterrents—to going down on your partner is fear that your gag reflex will kick in. This is especially true in deep throating situations, where the penis goes as far back as the throat and openings of the windpipe and esophagus. This issue can, with practice, remedy itself, with fellatio becoming easier over time. But what can you do if it doesn't?

Sex Q & A
Is it healthy to use oral sprays or oral sex mints for deep throating?
Novelty products like Go Deep Oral Spray and Go Deep Oral Sex Mints are products formulated with small amounts of benzocaine, which relaxes and numbs the throat muscles. While they promise longer, deeper oral sex, they should be used with caution. In containing this mild anesthetic, they reduce your throat sensations, diminishing your ability to detect when your body is taking on more than it can handle. Remember, your gag reflex is there for a reason, and using products like these can compromise your safety.

First and foremost, it's important to stress that your gag reflex isn't a bad thing. This auto-response to choking is normal; it's there to keep you breathing and to save your life. Whether it's due to food, an object, or someone's penis, your gag reflex is activated when something comes into contact with nerves at the back of your mouth and soft palate.

Convulsions and throat constriction ensue, causing your stomach to tighten and lurch, which is why you feel queasy.

When this happens during oral sex, stay cool, calm, and relaxed all over. In avoiding gagging while going down on him in the future, consider practicing any of the following tactics:

1. While not advisable, given your gag reflex is what it is for a reason, some people gently and carefully stick a finger down their throat, in hopes of reconditioning this reaction. While it invites the urge to purge at first, over time, this can reduce the gag trigger.
2. Practice with a dildo (or an object that won't break and possibly choke you). Hold the dildo at its base and insert it into your mouth, mimicking the gentle in-out motion used during fellatio. Don't rush, leisurely pushing the dildo farther back into your mouth a little more each time.

During actual fellatio, you can:

• Change the angle of pleasuring.
• Mentally distract yourself.
• Take a breather by backing off, maintaining strokes with your hand, and taking a few deep breaths before resuming.
• Find a rhythm, namely exhaling before the penis thrusts inward, and inhaling as you take it out.
• Keep the penis in the shallow part of your mouth until any gagging sensations pass.

Finally, you don't need to take your lover's entire penis into your mouth. There's plenty of pleasuring to be had without choking on his member. Even if you're determined to be a sword swallower, know that it's okay to take a break on occasion, surfacing to spend more time on the head of the penis or to suck on his scrotum. In any case, use your hand to control his movements and guide the depth of the penis, as well as the speed. You may also want to experiment with various sexual positions in testing shallow penetration preferences.

Jaw and Tongue Fatigue

You're licking. You're sucking. You're flicking. You're massaging. You're tired. Whether you have tongue fatigue, neck pains, sore mouth, or the dreaded jaw lock, you're cramping up and feel like you've had your fill of penis. But there's a partner to be pleasured, and you want to be a trooper. But how do you deal with a mouth losing its motor? Pursue any of the following:

- Practice jaw-strengthening exercises, e.g., chew gum regularly.
- Try using a different area of your tongue or let your lower lip go solo in providing stimulation.
- Pace yourself. Ideally, you'd be doing this to avoid the situation, but should it strike, resume a slow and steady pace.
- Carefully use your fingers to mimic your tongue until you feel recovered.
- Use Head Candy. This oral sex enhancement is candy pressed against your teeth to provide a soft, slippery cushion. It reduces jaw fatigue, protects your lover's loins from your teeth, and prevents dry mouth while increasing pleasure for the giver and receiver.

In further dealing with mouth or body fatigue, ways to maintain the action while taking a break include:

- Incorporate a vibrator to maintain hot spot stimulation.
- Use your fingers.

- Mix up techniques for variety.
- Change rhythms.

Sex Q & A

How can fellatio be made easier when going down on a well-endowed man?

Women who perform oral sex on larger men often complain that their gag reflex kicks in when the penis goes too deep. In avoiding this reaction, stay relaxed, focusing on your breathing and performing oral sex in a position where you feel in control, e.g., he's on his back, with you over him. As you take him more deeply into your mouth, wrap a hand around his shaft and have it slide up and down his penis in unison with your mouth, keeping things well lubricated with saliva. This will give him the illusion of going completely into your mouth while making sure you're not choking on his member.

| Common Concerns for Him

While it is generally assumed that all men are perfectly fine with oral sex, your partner can be afflicted with issues that hold him back from becoming an oral sex enthusiast. If you're going down on your man and he's not as into it as you think he should be, don't take it personally. Here are some of the major issues your guy could be dealing with:

A Misbehaved Penis

Maybe your guy loves oral sex, but is afraid that his penis isn't going to cooperate. He fears losing his erection or getting off too early, either of which could be based on past negative experiences. While erectile dysfunction (ED) and premature ejaculation (PE) problems can be physiologically based, they're often psychologically rooted as well. Issues at hand can include: stress, depression, anger, lack of desire, frustration, distraction, unresolved partner conflict (including those involving exes), death, and not feeling mentally aroused.

The Solution: In avoiding problems with erectile functioning during oral sex, your lover should practice using condoms while masturbating. He should approach his self-pleasuring experience as though he's with a partner, mentally walking himself through the action. With practice, this will help him in developing his comfort level with a partner, building his confidence and ability to remain erect. This effort, however, needs to be complemented by addressing the emotional issues going on.

His erection (or lack thereof) lets both of you know that he's not totally comfortable with the sexual situation he's pursuing or the relationship he's in. This could be because he has not healed from his last relationship, because he's afraid of being burned again, or because oral sex is more intimate for him than you expected.

There's a great deal of vulnerability involved in your partner letting you take his penis into your mouth, even when he trusts you. It can be incredibly hard for your guy to relax and let himself surrender to having his sexual response in the spotlight. He may fear making noise, getting too active, emitting fluid, or simply being the star of the show. This may stem from negative messages he received about sex growing up, messages he was taught about what it means to be a "man" (in other words, always in control), or that he's not emotionally comfortable with the sex play at hand. Your partner may need more time to get to know you. For some people, it takes weeks and months to feel connected enough to fully enjoy oral sex. So allow yourselves the time, delaying gratification for greater pleasure and easier performance later.

"When receiving oral sex, the fact that she swallows eagerly is critical to emotional satisfaction. To me it means she accepts the most personal and intimate part of me (my seed) into her mouth and belly (from deep inside of me to deep inside of her)." } Gianni

Premature Ejaculation

A male can experience premature ejaculation (PE) at any point in his life. It's mostly psychological in nature, most commonly attributed to anxiety and often occurring during first experiences with sex. The amount of sex you have can also be a factor. The longer the period of time since he last ejaculated, the quicker your man will typically reach orgasm. Some men develop a long-term anxiety toward oral sex, which can cause a prolonged experience with premature ejaculation.

The Solution: Every man develops his own method for dealing with premature ejaculation. Some men use condoms to dull the senses in their penis long enough to avoid premature ejaculation. Some men masturbate before going on a date so that they'll be less aroused when, and if, they engage in sex. The majority of men with PE learn to control their orgasms and ejaculatory responses by practicing Kegel exercises for males, which work the pelvic floor muscles. This is coupled with a male becoming incredibly familiar with every aspect of his sexual response.

To prevent premature ejaculation, your guy needs to learn to recognize the ejaculation sensations that occur just before he's about to ejaculate—that "point of inevitability" when he can't stop his orgasm or ejaculation. The next time you go down on him, have him tune into the sensations, and just as he starts to reach this point, pull back. Stop all stimulation so that his ejaculatory response isn't triggered. Once he's "come down" a bit, resume stimulation, stopping again when you're about to reach that "point of ejaculatory inevitability." Let him know what you're doing so that he doesn't assume that you're just being a tease.

Sex Savvy

To avoid early ejaculation, perform the Squeeze Technique. As he nears the point of ejaculatory inevitability, you or he should squeeze and apply pressure on the penis using your thumb and one or two of your forefingers, either at the base of the penis or at the ridge under the head.

Condom Use

A big reason for the lack of condom use during fellatio is that some males fear the dulled sensation will cause them to lose their erections.

The Solution: Encourage your guy to practice using condoms while he masturbates, getting used to the process and the sensations experienced with this type of stimulation. He should approach his self-pleasuring experience as though you are performing oral sex on him, mentally picturing the seduction, including the "pause" that's needed for protection, to your mouth wrapping itself around his shaft to your lips massaging the length of his shaft with every oral thrust. With practice (and getting used to the latex), this will help your guy develop his comfort level for condoms.

Oral Sex Inhibitions

Whether as giver or receiver, people have lots of hang-ups about oral sex for a number of different reasons. In some cases, these can make it difficult to relax and let go and experience the "big O." For others, inhibitions make for an oral phobia, with fellatio viewed as dirty, taboo, or a total turn-off. Some of these can be alleviated in getting to know your partner and feeling comfortable together. A supportive, healthy, loving relationship can do wonders for any oral sex issues. Yet regardless of one's relationship situation, there are situations that can lend themselves to a strong dislike or disgust of oral sex.

Psychological Control

Sex is a head game more than anything, with your pleasuring boiling down to what's going on between your ears more than what's happening between your legs. Your mind can play games when it comes to oral efforts, especially if you've been raised with negative messages about oral sex as dirty or wrong. Research has found, for example, that negative religious beliefs about oral sex restrain such sexual activity.

Reasons for the need to maintain psychological control during sex vary greatly, and may need to be explored with a certified sex therapist or counselor depending on the issues at hand. In the meantime, if your state of mind is controlling your ability to embrace oral, you need to learn to let go and replace negative thoughts with positive sexual affirmations. For example, your partner can replace an anti-oral thought with, "I deserve this kind of pleasure. It is wonderful and I will let myself succumb to it." Or, when psyching yourself up to give, you can formulate a mantra for yourself, such as "Oral sex is good for my mind, body, soul, and relationship. I will let it be so." Practice it on a regular basis.

Rolls Off the Tongue

"It's such a stereotype that guys can get hard or cum any time they can get action. I've found that if I'm not comfortable with the situation, the girl, or the relationship, I'm suddenly dealing with ED, premature ejaculation, or delayed ejaculation. My body just doesn't want to work with me and I've finally accepted that it's trying to tell me that something's wrong with what's going on—at least for me." }Dan

Sexual Abuse

It's very common for people—men and women—who have been sexually violated to suffer from sexual repercussions later in life, though this is not the rule. Touch or certain sex acts can trigger memories and sensations resembling the abuse, stirring up feelings that majorly interfere with pleasure. Survivors may avoid or fear sex, see it as an obligation, experience negative feelings with touch, have trouble with arousal or feeling sensation, or feel distance or not be present, among a whole host of other difficulties. The after effects of the trauma include fear, disempowerment, and distress, all of which shut down sexual response and interest. When sexual intimacy is managed, a survivor may experience numbness from unwanted touch. It's not uncommon for a person to avoid sex or see it as an obligation, which kills any enjoyment to be had.

In healing from this ultimate violation of trust, affection, and privacy, a survivor needs to seek therapy and sexual healing, which involve reconnecting with the body in positive ways, e.g., bubble baths and relearning touch exercises. These activities involve couples sharing love, respect, and appreciation. This process of reclaiming one's sexuality as pleasurable and positive also involves introspective work, increased awareness of the self and body, developing positive attitudes toward sexuality, and acquiring new skills for touch and sexual sharing. It can take months or years, and is best done under the guidance of a counselor or therapist specializing in supporting survivors.

| Overcoming Sexual Aversions to Oral Sex

An aversion is an unconscious, negative physiological and emotional reaction due to a person having had bad experiences with a behavior or extremely unpleasant emotional experience. A person with an aversion has learned to associate those bad experiences or feelings with a task or situation, and, hence, has been conditioned to react at the mere thought of "X" with anxiety, distress, and unhappiness. Aversions can also stem from lovers trying to meet each other's emotional and sexual needs if this effort is associated with an unpleasant experience. These typically stem from a partner becoming physically and/or emotionally abusive, including putting pressure on a lover, or being very sensitive when a need isn't met to his or her satisfaction.

Sexual aversion can get to the point that engaging in sex acts one wants to avoid can suppress sexual response or make arousal and orgasm unpleasant when they occur. Symptoms include a fear of engaging in sexual intimacy, attempts to make the sex act as short as possible, trying to find excuses to avoid or postpone sexual intimacy, feeling ill and/or depressed just before or after sex, and needing to build up your confidence before sexual activity just to get through it. The experience is more of a panic attack than anything, with some actually experiencing such during intimacy.

For you or your lover to overcome an aversion, you must break the association of sex with the unpleasant emotional reaction and associate it with a state of relaxation. This begins with learning how to relax when you think about sex. Set aside fifteen minutes a day to sit by yourself, comfortably, and think about the experiences you have had. Notice the feelings that come up. Now, instead of thinking about sex, redirect your thoughts to relaxing experiences, making an attempt to relax different muscle groups in your body. Start from the feet and slowly work your way up, giving yourself time to unwind. Once relaxed, think about sex again, only staying totally relaxed. Don't think about the specific sex issue causing you distress, but imagine different aspects of sex, like your fantasies, noting your reactions. What acts hold appeal? Which ones do not? Remember to stay relaxed.

Write down what you learned about yourself. Which thoughts made it difficult versus easy to relax? Work through the ones causing you distress in future fifteen-minute timeouts. Eventually, you'll want to learn how to relax at the thought of oral sex. Your goal is to stop the unpleasant reactions from occurring when presented with the situation. You can do this by relaxing at the thought of it, "extinguishing" the aversive association. Eventually, you'll want to relax yourself head to toe before an attempt to engage in oral sex. Note the feelings that come up as you relax your way through negative emotions. These may prevent you from "going all the way" all at once and may take more than one attempt. Challenge yourself, but not to the point you're causing yourself distress. Once you have learned to relax at the thought of oral sex, see what you're capable of—and only after you and your partner have an understanding that you're the one in charge.

If your partner doesn't reciprocate, keep your efforts sincere. If you give in order to receive, and not out of like or love, then that's not going to help your cause. People tend to pick up on that energy and shut down. Oral sex shouldn't be used as a trade-off or investment in your ultimate pleasuring.

Health and Relationship Benefits

Knowing the health benefits of oral sex can be a great excuse to get down to business. Sex, in general, is loaded with health and relationship benefits when your interactions with another are positive, informed, and practiced safely. And it's not simply the sexologists and health advocates who are hailing the wonders of sex. Even economists have claimed that regular sex can bring people as much happiness as would a $50,000/year raise. The more sex, it's said, the happier the individual.

Sex Q & A

Is it okay to kiss your lover after giving oral sex?

While some lovers have no problem with locking lips after oral sex, others will have nothing of it. Some people see this as a very intimate act and a testament to their bond in sharing everything, while others think it's gross, especially if emission was involved. To kiss or not to kiss post-oral really comes down to your and your partner's preferences. So be sure to talk about it and cases where it's hot versus not.

Oral sex, in a safe context, can be a source of physical, psychological, and spiritual well-being. It can enhance your mind, body, and soul, offering the following:

- Stress relief. Being sexually active counters body tension, with sexual response releasing the cuddle hormone oxytocin into your system. Oxytocin stimulates feelings of warmth and relaxation, bolstering your ability to respond to stress.
- Greater intimacy. Oral sex can make for a stronger, longer-lasting relationship, enhancing the intimacy experienced between you and your partner.
- Better sleep. Sleep is the foundation of all health, with the orgasms attained from oral sex enabling you to catch some zzzz's more easily.
- Pick me ups. Oral sex can boost your mood, with elevated arousal and orgasm-releasing, pleasure-inducing endorphins that can relieve depression and anxiety and up vitality.

It cannot be stated enough: Sexual fulfillment is a critical component of one's quality of life and health. Oral sex is one form of sexual intimacy that can help you to realize your life to the fullest, making you a more connected lover and part of a happier relationship.

| Common Myths

Despite the wealth of information now available about sex, largely thanks to the Internet, there's a lot of misinformation out there as well. People have been fed myths about oral sex since their youth, with these misconceptions often impacting their willingness to engage in oral pleasuring, for better or for worse. Preconceptions and myths about oral sex are major deterrents for those who haven't tried it. The following are some of the most common myths and the real-deal rebuttals:

MYTH	REAL DEAL
You can get pregnant from swallowing ejaculate.	Absolutely not!
There's only one easy way to send your partner into bliss.	Every individual is different when it comes to oral sex preferences and what it takes to help them to reach climax. This can also vary from one sex session to the next. The only way to find out how to launch your lover into the cosmos is to ask what's working—how things feel—during and after sex.
Rubbing or swallowing ejaculate can clear up acne and menstrual cramps, give you bigger breasts, and whiten your teeth.	Males have been known to come up with some goodies to get their partner to swallow. But all of these fallacies are just that—wrong!
All men want their partner to swallow.	While some men would really like for their lover to swallow their semen, others are totally indifferent, while others would rather that you not. Find out what your lover's thoughts are on the matter!
When you go down on your partner, you run the risk of your partner peeing in your mouth with climax.	This is virtually impossible, but if at some point, you come into contact with your own or your partner's urine, realize that it's mostly water and relatively sterile. It's harmless as long as it doesn't get into an orifice or wound, as this could transmit infection.

Whether you or your lover find yourselves still troubled by any of these issues, consider consulting a sex educator, counselor, therapist, or coach. Sometimes simply talking to somebody or getting reassurances about your concerns can be liberating. Such services can also help you to counter one of the biggest hang-ups about oral sex: genital perceptions because how people see themselves can hugely impact how much oral they're up for and just how much they'll let themselves enjoy it.

CHAPTER 9

Genital Perceptions: Attending to the Senses

He longs to let you go down on him, but he has deep-seeded concerns about his genitals. Trust me, he's not alone. A number of people wonder if they're normal or if there's something wrong going on down there. People are reluctant to receive oral sex for a number of reasons, with lack of body confidence and knowledge about their genitals major barriers to such sexual pursuits. Many are worried about whether they smell or taste bad. Some fret over whether or not their genitals are unsightly. Some stress over the potential of performance issues, like problems with attaining erection, given personal issues they have with what's between their legs. This is so unfortunate given the attitude you—and your partner—have toward your genitals is an important component of your sexual experiences and your ability to let go and fully enjoy yourself.

Genital Perceptions

A study in the *Journal of Sex Research* reported that favorable perceptions of one's genitalia not only correlate positively with engaging in
sexual activities, like oral sex, but enjoying such as well. How your
partner feels about his private parts may, in fact, be more important
than how he feels about his look overall. One study conducted at Old
Dominion University found that perceptions of the body during sexual
activity may be more influential on one's sexual functioning than the
self-assessment of one's physical appearance. In addition, individuals
who are content with their bodies also report more sex and are likelier
to attain orgasm.

Sex Savvy

A review of letters from women to Indiana University's Kinsey Institute for Sex, Gender & Reproduction revealed that
penis size inquiries typically involved the complaint of a
lover being too big. Letter writers feared that their lover might
hurt them.

While recent years have seen a lot of efforts focus on boosting
female perceptions of their genitals, not nearly as much has been done
for males. Can your guy say that he has made friends with his genitals? Men are often really hard on themselves when it comes to what's
below-the-belt, flustered that they don't look perfect down there. And
your guy won't even feel perfect if he's comparing himself to the altered
and airbrushed visuals of waxed, makeup-covered, and even surgically
manipulated genitalia portrayed in porn magazines and flicks. Ironi-
cally, nobody looks like those porn stars, including the models themselves. Yet many of us are guilty of holding everyone up to unrealistic,
unattainable standards!

His "Look"

When it comes to the penis, no two are the same, with the vast majority nowhere near the "third leg" erections flaunted by porn stars. Studies have suggested that viewing sexually explicit material contributes to men rating their penises as smaller than average. Ultimately, the social and psychological consequences, like low self-confidence, sexual anxiety, fear of relationships, and social maladjustment, can wreak havoc in the bedroom and in relationships.

What guys need to realize is that penises come in a host of shape and size combinations when flaccid or erect. The same goes for balls, with one side often hanging lower or slightly larger than the other. Yet many men are obsessed over the size of their penises, convinced that they need to be well hung. Others are self-conscious about whether their nuts look normal. Add to that the misinformation and stereotypes circulating about the penis when it comes to performance and you have many men harshly judging themselves.

The most ironic and troubling thing about this issue is the fact that the perfect size penis is itself an illusion. The vast majority of men are "average," or within 2 inches of the average length, which falls at 3–4 inches in length for a flaccid (nonerect) penis, and 5–7 inches in length for an erect penis. While many men think that they have a micropenis (a penis that is less than 3 inches erect), this condition affects only 0.6 percent of men. Most men afflicted with "small penis syndrome," a.k.a. "locker room syndrome," actually have average-sized members.

Unbelievably, despite no reliable data regarding the criteria for success or complications of penile enlargement procedures, between 1991 and 1998, 10,000 men in the United States paid thousands of dollars to undergo penile augmentation. One unpublished study at New York University found that men who described themselves as having large genitalia had a more favorable genital image, body image, and beliefs about their sexual abilities than those men who saw their genitals as average or small in size. While this is great for men who feel that they're well-endowed, this is a shame for men who beat themselves up for not being hung like a horse, especially when you consider that most women don't care about the size.

Sex Savvy

There is no safe way to permanently enlarge the penis. While penile surgery is an option, it can potentially cause damage and performance problems. With girth enhancement, the fat that is injected into the penis may not take, resulting in a lumpy, swollen looking, mutated organ with a distorted shape. In lengthening the penis, the release of the penile suspensory ligament, which detaches it from the lower abdomen, can cause problems as well—primarily an erection that fails to salute. Tell your lover that the next time he daydreams about becoming the next Ron Jeremy!

Judging Genitals

Some women have been known to judge their partner's genitals based on unfair societal standards. Not knowing any better, they get turned off that their guy doesn't look like the latest *Playgirl* centerfold. It's important to remember that every guy is different and beautifully unique when it comes to what's between his legs. That's part of what makes every individual sexy and enticing. Bigger, smaller, thinner, fatter, longer, shorter . . . your guy needs to embrace what Mother Nature has given him; he needs to work on his self-confidence instead of trying to fix something that isn't broken. He needs to learn to love and appreciate the gems he has between his legs if he ever expects to awaken their full potential. The pay-offs are huge!

Research in the *Electronic Journal of Human Sexuality* examining the genital perceptions of Canadian college students found that men had consistently more favorable views of their genitals than did women. Males and females who had had intercourse further reported more favorable genital perceptions than did virgins. Self-esteem was positively correlated to favorable genital perceptions, and negatively with sexual anxiety and feeling self-conscious about one's body. For those experiencing genital dissatisfaction, penis size was the main issue for men.

So take the time to sit down with your guy and appreciate his body; get to know what gives his genitals character and highlight what you like about them. This could be his penis's color, shape, folds, plumpness, protrusions, and so on. Ask him to do the same for your parts. Remember, what's normal is to be different and your partner's ability to respond sexually and experience and share pleasure has nothing to do with the way he looks, but how well he can embrace his sexual self in its entirety. You can support him in this by letting him know that you're perfectly happy with what he has.

Sex Savvy

A review of sixty years of research in the *British Journal of Urology* assessed that penis length matters more to men than women, with 90 percent of women preferring a wide penis to a long one. The same review reported that 85 percent of women were satisfied with their partner's penis size versus only 55 percent of men having no qualms with their own.

When He's *Au Naturel*— The Uncircumcised Penis

Most men around the world are uncircumcised, meaning their penises are intact; their foreskins have not been removed. For the past few decades, the majority of infant males in the United States have been circumcised, though this is changing. With the uncircumcised fellow still the exception to the rule, however, women are often surprised or taken aback, at least initially, in dealing with his "extra" part. For some, it's a matter of aesthetics. For others, there's a concern over how to play with his foreskin during oral sex, especially given that this delicate area is packed with nerve endings and must be handled with care.

Rolls Off the Tongue

"My father challenged the doctor who wanted to snip me as an infant, telling him to leave my foreskin intact—or else. I will be eternally grateful. While some people make a big deal out of being circumcised, I feel lucky to still have all of my parts. The foreskin is an amazing erogenous zone. I wish that more people would see it as that instead of a hygienic issue. I'm certainly cleaner than a lot of men who are cut, probably because I give my penis extra attention in the shower!" } Sam

Personal preferences aside, once you're comfortable with the foreskin, there's plenty of fun to be had with this highly sensitive thin layer of skin. If you're having trouble with the fact that he's uncut, educate yourself on the myths that run rampant about the uncircumcised penis. For example, an uncircumcised penis is just as clean as its circumcised brothers when washed on a daily basis.

Learn, too, about the potential sex play, and in some cases better sex, to be had with Mother Nature's original form. If you're turned off by the look, realize that the foreskin typically retracts over the shaft, exposing the head of the penis when your lover is erect, giving him a more circumcised look. This "sleeve" acts like a natural lubricant during all types of sex, gliding in its bed of movable skin so that chafing is minimized, while providing both partners with pleasurable friction.

Sex Savvy

In cases where the foreskin doesn't completely retract when erect, gently pull down on it, using your fingertips or tongue, to uncover the head. This is best done by first moistening the area with lube or saliva. Check in with your partner to learn just how far back the foreskin can go and still feel good. Find out how he likes to be touched, asking him to point out the most reactive hot spots along his shaft.

| Passion amidst Pubic Hair

People sport all sorts of "looks" when it comes to their pubic hair, with color, amount, and texture varying greatly. Some go completely bare, while others strive for a specific style and others keep what Mother Nature gave them. For lovers pursuing passion amidst pubes, getting a hair stuck in your throat can happen, causing much discomfort and distress to those who have been there. So how do you avoid this hairy situation? The easiest way involves combing through your lover's pubic hair with your fingers ahead of time. Massage his pubic area prior to going south as a part of foreplay, shaking loose any stragglers that could try to trump your game.

If the hair down there continues to be a problem—or if you're of the opinion that less is more—suggest hair removal as a form of foreplay or a sexy intimate session in and of itself. You can spend a leisurely afternoon or evening with your lover removing his hair, and pampering him with a sensual bath and erotic massage to boot. Hair removal can be as simple as a good trim of the hair covering the pubic bone using manicuring scissors, to snipping the hair around or on the scrotum, to shaving, waxing, tweezing, or using depilatories along the bikini line. Have fun experimenting with different looks on occasion, and even color, given that, no matter what the form of hair removal, your partner's pubes almost always grow back, albeit itchy and uncomfortably initially.

Rolls Off the Tongue

"More than anything—guy or gal—I think it's important to look like you have a well-maintained bush. It doesn't matter how much or how little hair you have down there, just as long as it's clean and well-groomed."

}Kai

Smell: P.U. vs. Passion-Inducing

Every one of us has a distinctive "signature scent," and we would perhaps do a better job embracing this natural aphrodisiac if it weren't for the smell-like-roses messaging we're bombarded with regularly. As you probably well know, sweating can cause a stronger genital odor. People can minimize unpleasant smells by avoiding synthetic (polyester) underwear and Spandex clothes that do not allow the genitals to breathe. Cotton underwear and exercise clothes, as well as loose clothes in general, are best in circulating air around the groin. Otherwise, bacteria can further set up shop, growing in a sweaty environment that causes undesirable odors.

The odor of your partner's sweat can also be influenced by his diet, so if smell is a problem, mention that he avoid consuming too much sugar, caffeine, and alcohol. No matter what he does, tell him not to use deodorants of any sort down there since these are not made for use on the mucous membranes of the genitals and may have chemicals that can irritate and cause an undesirable reaction.

If your partner is his own worst critic with his scent, or thinks that he doesn't need to do things like shower after he comes home from the gym and wants you all over him, it's time for a reality check. He needs to be realistic in his expectations. It's humanly impossible to always be "shower fresh," but most people prefer that their lovers maintain a certain level of cleanliness. So be sure to highlight the moments you think his genital region smells oh-so-good.

His Personal Scent

Men need to be mindful about washing their genitals daily with warm water and soap. If your guy is uncircumcised, you may notice a distinct scent when getting up close and personal to his genitals. This is normal, even when he washes under his foreskin daily. The foreskin's sebaceous glands secrete emollients, lubricants, and protective antibodies that help to keep the surface of the tip of the penis soft and moist. A strong odor may just require a wash with a gentle, antibacterial soap, especially if there's a build-up of smegma, the fatty matter that collects between the glans and foreskin. This is not only important because of dirt and bacteria build up, which can have his penis smelling and tasting bad, but it decreases your risk of acquiring an STD. For any male, redness, irritation, or an offensive odor, among other unusual symptoms, may indicate an infection, e.g., yeast infection. Be sure to recommend that your guy is checked out by a healthcare provider if that's the case.

Sex Savvy

If you think that your partner could use some freshening up, suggest taking a shower together as a form of foreplay, perhaps with the lights off to encourage becoming even more uninhibited.

Taste

When you initially go down on your guy, unless you're using protection, your taste buds are likeliest to detect some degree of saltiness, though he may taste tangier or muskier at times. A guy's taste most often boils down to his sweat and discharge, which is in part dependent upon his diet. Garlic and onions, for example, can result in strong odors that influence taste. His taste can also come down to what you're used to. If you have a diet high in soy sauce, for example, you may not pick up on salty influences on bodily fluids as much as those who only use it on occasion.

The taste of a man's semen can be a turn-off if he is a smoker, has been drinking, or recently consumed asparagus, broccoli, or curry. To make sure he's appetizing, he should avoid these products, as well as coffee, beets, cauliflower, red meat, fish, and vitamins for twenty-four hours prior to sex if possible to neutralize the scent of his ejaculate as scent ties strongly into how things taste. Have him try consuming celery and parsley instead. Furthermore, he should drink lots of water and sweeten his cum by consuming melons, blueberries, pineapple juice, lemon, cranberry, pineapple, raspberries, and strawberries. Cardamom, cinnamon, and peppermint are also said to make him tastier.

At the end of the day, your lover needs to experiment with his diet to see how it affects his semen. This not only includes the foods and beverages themselves, but the amount consumed. If he's concerned about the way he tastes, he may want to taste his ejaculate the next time he masturbates or the next time the two of you fool around (provided he's in good sexual health). Ultimately, however, just how yummy he is comes down to your palate, which you can't be faulted for.

Sex Q & A
Is it a good idea to have an enema before engaging in analingus?
Prior to rimming, some people use a mild enema, which involves releasing water into the anus to trigger a bowel movement or to rid the anal cavity of feces and bacteria. When injecting liquid into the rectum and colon, use gentle products to avoid irritation or any cuts that could lead to infection. Enemas should also be performed infrequently since they may disrupt the body's eliminating process, as well as the rectum, bowels, and gastrointestinal tract.

| To Spit or Swallow
Spit versus swallow preferences vary from lover to lover and from one sex session to the next. Some women are perfectly happy to have a guy ejaculate in their mouths and have no problem with swallowing. Others, however, are not keen on either activity.

Despite there being a wide range of preferences on this matter, the "spit or swallow" debate rages on. This is in large part because swallowing semen is often ranked highly on the intimacy scale. It's seen as a form of bonding and a test of devotion and love, with some lovers putting pressure on a lover to receive in an effort to feel closer. If this describes your relationship, know that taking someone's sperm into your mouth is not a testament of love. Not wanting to do so, does not mean that you don't care about him.

There are a number of reasons why people choose not to swallow a partner's semen. They may not like the taste or texture, and worry about gagging or throwing up. They may be concerned about acquiring a sexually transmitted infection. Or they may be hesitant in not knowing what they're swallowing (over 95 percent of semen is water) or want the extra calories (your average ejaculation has 10–30 calories).

To spit or swallow is a question that should be answered before you go down on your guy. If you don't want him to ejaculate in your mouth, let him know ahead of time so that he can withdraw or let you know when he's close to ejaculation. If you don't want him ejaculating in your mouth, you have several options in helping him to peak following withdrawal:

- Switch to intercourse, either well before he's about to unload or right before the critical moment.
- Masturbate him to finish him off.
- Have him ejaculate into a towel or on you.

If you'd like to try swallowing, but dislike the taste of semen, have a chaser within arm's reach, like ice tea or Coca Cola.

Rolls Off the Tongue

"I don't swallow for just anybody. It has to be somebody that I'm involved with, love, and want to pleasure like no other. I also have to be in the mood to gulp and have the stomach for it. There are a number of factors that can play into whether or not his semen is appetizing, like how recently he ejaculated, what he's had to eat, and how my stomach is feeling." }Hunter

If your partner has finished in your mouth, but you don't want to swallow, have tissues or towel close by for a discreet one-tablespoon spit. Alternatively, you can make a quick beeline for the bathroom sink or engage in snowballing, where you kiss it right back to its owner.

At the end of the day, no matter what a pair's issues, lovers need to talk. That's why Chapter 10 is packed full of suggestions on how to get this type of sex talk going. Opening your mouths for the other type of oral can end up being some of the most intimate, erotic action you'll ever see (or hear).

Opening Your Mouth for Oral the Other Way: Sex Communication

Perhaps second best to having oral sex is talking about it with somebody you love to orally adore. Whether dealing with issues related to oral sex or wanting to discuss ways to change up or further eroticize oral, talking confidently about sex is often what elevates the action to another level. Lovers in healthy relationships engage in sex talks that allow them to avoid or resolve sexual issues and relationship dilemmas, or take sexual experiences to a whole new level. Talking about likes, dislikes, fears, shames, fantasies, and your emotional connection to your lover can help you to learn about your own and your partner's beliefs, shaping your experiences and evoking greater feelings.

Talking about Oral Sex

For some people, talking about oral sex is a fairly easy endeavor. They can unabashedly discuss their desires, needs, feelings, and difficulties. They can also listen to such sharings without squirming. Yet being sexually expressive and responsive isn't easy for most. Most people aren't given opportunities to talk about their sexual beliefs, attitudes, and values in a safe space. Most people are not raised with healthy role models when it comes to good communication, let alone savvy sex communication. Making matters all the more difficult are negative reactions lovers can have when the topic of oral sex is touched upon. Many times people become not only terribly uncomfortable and physically and emotionally withdrawn, but critical, judgmental, and even verbally abusive in projecting their discomfort and upset.

It's important for lovers to share and ask about one's wants around oral sex, as well as any difficulties in giving or receiving. In having these conversations, you and your partner need to be mindful about keeping yourselves in check, releasing any negative judgments, and seeking to be patient with each other in overcoming any difficulties. Thankfully, there are rules of engagement that lovers can strive to abide by in making their efforts less stressful.

Rolls Off the Tongue

"In some ways, while the most difficult, our conversations about sex are the best ones we have because we try so hard to be effective communicators. This forces us to be more vulnerable in what we reveal and more careful with what we say. Even if we stumble, the extra effort we put into these talks highlights how much we care about each other." } Rae

Rules of Engagement

In striving for respectful communication, it's important to realize that you're responsible for how you act and react. In taking responsibility for your role, and in having conversations marked by openness, acceptance, and appreciation, you will really listen for what's being said. With affection and compassion, reflect—and take steps—to make sure that each other's points are understood. You can do this in making sure that the following guidelines steer your efforts:

- Have talks when you don't have to worry about any interruptions or distractions, and when you feel ready to give your undivided attention.
- Be sincere in stating your needs, wants, and limits, as this helps to cultivate your partner's sense of safety.
- Respect and support your lover, as this will help him to feel valued.
- Stay positive, avoid criticism, and think about what you're saying both verbally and nonverbally.
- Encourage more details with "Tell me more" or "I'm listening."
- Ask open-ended questions so that the response you get isn't so limited.
- Reflect back if you're not sure about what's being said, e.g., "Am I hearing you correctly in that you're saying . . . ?"
- Ask to take a break if you need one or ask if you can have some time to think about a matter before responding.
- Validate each other's feelings, e.g., "I didn't know that you felt thát way. Let's figure out what we can do about that."
- Reflect on what you're thinking and how that's making you feel and react.
- Thank your partner for sharing, stating that you're glad that you talked if you feel that way.

Remember, it doesn't help to change the subject; to dismiss the other's fears, worries, and desires; or act like a know-it-all. Don't interrupt, use absolutes like "never," or use sarcastic, hostile tones. Finally, don't push your lover to the edge when it comes to oral sex expectations—instead of getting turned on to your hopes, your lover will tune out. These sex talks can be intense, and you may have to have several of them on the same subject before feeling like you've made progress or fully shared and understand one another.

Initiating Oral Sex Talks

When initiating conversations about oral sex with a partner who hasn't been responsive to such sexual intimacy, request permission; for example, start by saying something like, "I've been thinking about oral sex and our sex life. Can we talk about it?" If your partner is unresponsive, you can still state how this lack of reaction makes you feel and your concerns as to how this reflects upon other issues in the relationship. If necessary, suggest that the two of you seek sex counseling or therapy, if only for having a safe space, with a mediator, in which to air out issues. No matter where you have these sex talks, go into the conversation with no expectations, including thinking that you're going to change a partner's behaviors or attitudes. Your hope should be to simply feel heard, satisfied that you gave the chance at oral intimacy a fair shot.

Whether or not oral sex is ever realized, constructive conversations about this sexual behavior can result in greater understanding and emotional intimacy. Your hopes of being truly heard will be made more successful if you try:

- Listening, as well as paraphrasing and using reinforcement in reflecting what's being said. Note: This doesn't mean that you are necessarily agreeing with your partner, but showing that you understand.

- Being attentive. Be engaged and ask helpful questions to show you're into the conversation.
- Showing appreciation for what's being communicated, e.g., "I really appreciate that you're taking the time to work this out with me . . ."
- Showing that you value your partner, even when you beg to differ on a matter, e.g., "You know that I care about you a lot, but I'm bothered that you . . ."
- Using self-disclosure.
- Highlighting any positives about the situation.
- Encouraging more conversation, e.g., "Keep talking to me."
- Being physically supportive, e.g., holding your partner's hand.
- Owning your statements with "I" instead of other pronouns.

Your Nonverbals

While we've been giving a lot of attention to what comes out of your mouth (and your partner's), we also need to pay attention to the nonverbal messages you're sending to your lover when talking about oral sex. So evaluate your efforts regarding the following:

- Your eye contact. Are you having trouble looking your partner directly in the eyes?
- Body language. Are you saying that you're open, or are your arms and legs crossed, making you appear closed off?
- Your facial expressions. Do you look stone cold or are you being expressive in reflecting your internal reactions?
- Your volume. Are you getting louder, indicating that you're nervous or uneasy?

| Decide Who's Doing What

There are times when one partner will want to take charge and please a lover to no end. Then there are times when sex is more mutually initiated and, once the ball gets rolling, who is doing what orally will be decided in seconds. Typically, people see the giver as active and submissive, and the receiver as passive and dominant. However, there's a lot more fluidity in the power dynamic between roles.

When you're going down on your man, you're very much in charge of the action. You're the one setting the pace, deciding upon the type of stimulation, and overall steering the sex. As a receiver, your lover is very much in charge of his reactions. This involves his ability to let go, as in get out of his head and immerse himself in the pleasuring he's receiving. It also involves both of you being able to ask for what you want, provide direction when desired, and to give affirmations on a job well done. Unless couples are in a relationship where there's a major power divide between partners, or they're having fun engaging in such role-play scenarios, lovers are very much sharing the power dynamic when oral sex is involved.

"The action isn't always seamless as far as who is doing what, which is the only part of oral sex that was a turn-off. So we developed a signal. If I plan to go down on him, I draw a line down his treasure trail, and vice versa if he plans to go down on me. It's cute because sometimes there's a rush to be the first to make the line, while other times, we'll keep the foreplay going and totally tease each other in wondering who is going to make the line first. It's fun torture since that usually means that both of us really want to have the other go down!" }Celia

| Feedback

In striving to give the best oral sex ever, you need to ask for guidance from your guy. In some cases, he may be perfectly content, and honestly not have any guidance to give. In other cases, especially while in the moment and with new lovers, your lover will share. So go ahead and ask about the type of motion preferred, e.g., "Do you like it when I move my tongue side to side or in circles?" Ask what erogenous zones need to be touched more. Encourage him to tell you when to stop action, perhaps because a hot spot can't handle any more stimulation, and then when to start again.

When getting reactions from your guy, your attitude should be one of "I want to learn" and "I long to please." Ask for information if it's needed, e.g., "Tell me about your . . ." or tell your lover what needs to be done in order for you to maximize your efforts, e.g., "Spread your legs even more." Or share what you're about to do or the reaction you're aiming for, e.g., "I'm going to make you. . . . " Go ahead and ask things like:

- "What do you want me to do right now?"

- "Do you want me to go harder? Softer? Faster? Slower?"
- "What do you need for me to do more than anything?"
- "Does that excite you?"

When processing your oral sex experience or renewed efforts, ask each other:

- "What was that like for you?"
- "Was there anything you would have liked for me to have done differently?"
- "Where could I have given you more (attention, feedback . . .)?"
- "Based on what we just did, what would you like for us to do differently next time?"

Sex Savvy

When you and your partner are talking about sex, give encouragement and show appreciation. Accept and enjoy compliments about your abilities as a lover and qualities as a partner when they're given.

If you're not getting the feedback you want, encourage your guy to open up to you; tell him that you're open to constructive criticism if it's needed. Ask him to share what's working or not, followed by a suggestion for improvement, e.g., "I like it when you touch me using that technique, only I'd love more pressure on my perineum." Tell him it's okay for him to ask you to "tease, grab, touch, or feel" something in a particular area. Your man shouldn't be afraid to say, "I want you to _____ my _____" or "I want you to play with my _____." Such guidance should always be well received.

Sex Q & A

How can you tell when a guy is about to cum?

While there are general sexual responses that most people experience as they approach peaking—which is almost always accompanied with ejaculation for guys—there is no sure way to tell if your lover is about to climax and ejaculate. If you're concerned about a partner's emissions during oral sex, ask that he give you a head's up to pull away before they release.

Keep Oral Sex Sexy

Sex communication involves a lot more than talking about oral sex. It's also about those sensual, romantic, or really racy things you and your lover say as you're getting it on. Depending on the mood you're after or what the moment calls for, you can add to the moment by being:

- Affectionate. Let him know how much he means to you with "I love you" or "I adore being intimate with you."
- Romantic. Woo your guy with "You look so handsome right now" or "It makes me so happy to see you smiling like that."
- Sensual. Put your lover at ease with flattery like: "You smell amazing" or "You look so sexy" or "Your taste totally turns me on." "Your _____ feels so _____ against my lips."
- Seductive. Super-charge foreplay with statements like: "Love your _____ and I can't wait to _____." "I want to taste more of you." "I can't wait to feel you in my mouth." "Does it make you hard when I lick you like this?" "Shall I continue?" "Are you ready for me to _____ you?"
- Dirty. Get raw and invite more XXX-action with lines like: "I want to feel you slide down my throat." "I want to suck you dry." "Pump faster/harder between my lips." "I can't wait to swallow it all."

If you're at a loss for words or don't feel like talking, keep in mind the power of sound. Moaning, groaning, gasping, screaming, sighing, wailing, whimpering, crying for joy, and so on are all wonderful sounds people make when expressing pleasure and ecstasy. Likewise, moments of silence can allow you and your lover to enjoy your sex sounds, like heavy breathing, the wetness, and rustling of sheets. Tuning into these sounds during oral sex can enhance sensations even more.

Rolls Off the Tongue

"Having a lover who is good at aural sex can make all of the difference in the world. If somebody is going down on you, you can increase enthusiasm in doing things like talking dirty. If you're giving, talking sexy gives you the excuse for a breather, while not killing the moment." } Nate

| Have Safer Sex

Do you think that oral sex is safer sex? Think again. As is the case with vaginal-penile and anal intercourse, engaging in fellatio poses sexual health risks that you need to think twice about. You and your lover need to take care of each other and your sexual and reproductive health by minimizing the risks involved in your oral fixation pursuits. It's not only the right thing to do, but can make everything even sweeter.

Rolls Off the Tongue

"I finally hooked up with a really babelicious friend, but had trouble enjoying myself as I went down on him knowing his ex-girlfriend had trouble with HPV. I couldn't get past worries like could he be a carrier? Could he be infecting me? I've been avoiding his interest in getting together again, for fear of putting myself at risk." } Carrie

Sexually Transmitted Infections

Sexually transmitted diseases (STDs), a.k.a. sexually transmitted infections (STIs), pose some degree of risk any time anybody engages in unprotected oral sex. If one partner's bodily fluids—semen (including pre-cum), vaginal fluid, blood, and/or breast milk—are infected, he or she runs the risk of infecting another with STDs like HIV, hepatitis, syphilis, gonorrhea, chlamydia, and nongonoccocal urethritis, during oral sex or other types of sexual activities.

Sex Savvy

If both partners are infected with HSV-1 (oral herpes) and HSV-2 (genital herpes), they cannot re-infect one another or cause the other more outbreaks, including when one partner has an active sore or is experiencing viral shedding. This is because the body has developed antibodies to both strains of the virus.

In other cases, STDs, like herpes, genital warts, scabies, and lice, may be transmitted simply via skin-to-skin contact. Confusing to many lovers is the matter of which STDs, like the herpes simplex virus strains, can be transferred from the mouth to the genitals and vice versa during oral sex.

Sex Savvy

A study of 300 people conducted by Johns Hopkins University found that the risk of throat cancer was nearly 9 times greater for people reporting oral sex with more than 6 partners.

During analingus, you run the additional risk of acquiring hepatitis A, lice, scabies, anal herpes, anal warts (HPV), parasitic infections, like amebiasis, and/or bacterial infections like e-coli. Kissing, licking, tonguing, or sucking on the anal opening with your lips and/or tongue invites the risk and spread of these harmful bacteria, viruses, and parasites, especially when exposed to anal cuts or tears or traces of bloody feces.

Being knowledgeable about the risks of oral sex can only work to your benefit, making you a more empowered lover in all that you do, or choose not to do. With worries about your sexual health put aside, you can allow yourself to become fully absorbed in the action. While a lot of what you're about to read may be hard to swallow (pun intended), you'll come away more sexually informed. It's hard to find thorough, accurate resources on this topic, so you only stand to heighten your bedroom rock star status in being completely in-the-know.

Rolls Off the Tongue

"I think I'd be more willing to give and receive oral sex if I felt more fully informed about the risks involved, as well as ways to protect myself. It's like people are afraid to talk about it because it's not sexy, which sounds ridiculous when you think of the consequences." } Marty

Factors That Increase Risk of Infection

When assessing the risk of acquiring an STD or passing one along, especially during unprotected oral sex, consider the following factors:

Active vs. Inactive Infection

While infections can be spread at any time, you want to avoid oral sex, or any kind of sex for that matter, when a partner has an outbreak, especially when either individual has open cuts or sores on or in the mouth or genitals.

Oral Health

If you're giving oral sex and have cuts, ulcers, bleeding gums, and sores in or around your mouth and throat, you're at increased risk of contracting an STD.

Dental Work

Related to your oral health is any recent dental work, including having undergone a root canal, having your wisdom teeth pulled, or getting dentures re-fitted. Going to the dentist for any kind of checkup or brushing or flossing your teeth before oral sexual activity also increases your risk of acquiring an STD. This is because these activities can result in lesions, scrapes, sores, irritations, or tiny cuts on the gums you may not even be aware of.

Sex Savvy

With early HIV research largely focusing on the anal sex practices of the homosexual community, scientists failed to pay enough attention to the oral transmission of HIV. A presentation of eight HIV cases, given at the Seventh Conference on Retroviruses and Opportunistic Infections, suggested that all of these cases were oral sex attributable, with all eight HIV-positive individuals having had some type of recent dental work.

Ejaculation

If you're performing oral sex and your partner ejaculates into your mouth, this increases your risk of infection. While it has yet to be confirmed, female ejaculation in one's mouth may also pose a threat.

STD Status

The presence of one STD increases the risk of acquiring another. So be sure to abstain, or at least practice safer sex, if either of you has an outbreak.

Sex Q & A

When suffering from a sore throat and swollen glands, how does a person know if he or she might have an STD versus simply have the start of strep throat or the common cold?

There is no way to tell with certainty if you acquired an infection during oral sex or if you're coming down with strep or a cold since these conditions often share many of the same symptoms, like fever, swollen glands, sore throat, and tonsillitis. Indicators that you may have an oral STD specifically include oral lesions or cold sores, though this is not a hard and fast rule. Symptoms may also last longer than your average sore throat or cold. In determining whether or not you have an STD, or just a cold, pay a visit to a healthcare professional, who will take a throat culture to determine the cause.

When to Play vs. When to Abstain

If you or your partner have an active STD, it practically goes without saying that it's best to abstain from sexual activity until the infection is treated or goes back to an inactive status. If your STD is curable, make sure that you refrain from sex until treatment is complete. Be sure to have your partner tested and treated as well. Failure to do so could result in you getting re-infected.

In cases where abstinence is out of the question or where a lover is carrying a lifelong, viral STD, safer sex options, as outlined in the next section, are available. You can further reduce the risk of transmission by having open, honest communication, limiting the number of sexual partners you have, and going for regular sexual and reproductive health checkups.

All of these points are really important given that many STDs are *asymptomatic* (without symptoms). A person can be a carrier and never even know that they're infected, especially since an infection may lie dormant in their systems for months or even years after exposure; they may not be aware that they pose a threat to others. Take, for example, the two-thirds of the 45 million Americans with genital herpes who never have any symptoms. Even when a person looks perfectly healthy, and the sexual exchange appears totally risk-free, make sure that you're both attuned to the need to discuss and employ safer sex practices.

Sex Savvy

Being on the birth control pill, or any other hormonal contraceptive, does not protect you or your partner from STDs—including HIV—during oral sex or other sexual activities.

Safer Sex Strategies

Aside from abstaining from sexual activity altogether, the only way to protect yourself from STDs is to use a male condom, female condom, dental dam, latex gloves, and/or finger cots, depending on your sex acts of choice. Here are prime ways to protect yourself and your lover:

Condoms

When it comes to oral sex, latex and polyurethane (plastic) condoms are recommended in decreasing the risk of STD transmission. As a sheath that's worn over an erect penis, the condom catches semen, preventing the spread of infection. While latex condoms are slightly more effective than polyurethane condoms, the latter is a great option for those with latex sensitivities or allergies. Polyurethane condoms are also thinner, allowing for greater heat transmission, sensitivity, and a nicer feel and appearance for some people. They are, though, less elastic and offer a looser fit, making them slightly more likely to slip off or break as you're getting busy.

In choosing a condom for oral sex, avoid ones that are lubricated since these may have a disgusting taste. Plain is best for your oral purposes, with Durex Clear Unlubricated, Trojan Enz, and Trojan Non-Lube among the name-brand latex condoms that can be slipped onto your guy's shaft for safer sex. Avanti Polyurethane is a nice tasteless option for those desiring plastic condoms. Note: Condoms are less effective in providing protection against HPV and herpes since these STDs can be spread via skin-to-skin contact.

Sex Savvy

The world's oldest surviving condom dates back to 1640. Made of pig intestines, it was used in Sweden, but its original user's manual was written in Latin. Unlike today's male condoms, it was possibly meant to be reusable. In preventing disease, the user was to soak the condom in warm milk first. Makes using today's prophylactics seem like a piece of cake!

Female Condoms

The female condom is a soft, polyurethane pouch which is inserted into the vagina prior to sex. It can also, though, be slipped over the penis during oral sex, especially as a great alternative for those with a latex allergy or sensitivity. Sold at select drug and grocery stores under brand names like Reality, Femidom, and Dominique, the inside of the condom is lined with a silicone-based lubricant for greater sensation. FC2 is the latest female condom, made out of nitrile, which makes it cheaper to produce.

Sex Savvy

Never use two condoms at the same time, including a female condom together with a male condom. This does not double your protection but rather creates more friction, making condom breakage likelier.

Flavored Condoms

Recommended for fellatio, flavored condoms that are FDA-approved for oral sex are a super way to spice up condom use. Lovers like the way the condom, or the lubes they contain, not only cover up the smell and taste of latex or plastic, but awaken the senses by enhancing taste and scent as well. Strawberry, banana, mint, grape, chocolate, orange, and vanilla flavors are just a smackering of the condoms you have to choose from, with trusted brands including Durex Flavored, Kiss of Mint (Lifestyles), and Trustex Flavored. Note: Novelty condoms that are edible are *not* good for protection against HIV or STDs (or pregnancy). As their label "For Novelty Use Only" implies, they are just for fun and variety. If that's all you're about, have a ball exploring assortments like champagne, chocolate, and lemon honey spritzer.

Dental Dams

A dental dam is a thin, square barrier, typically made out of latex, that provides protection against STDs, including HIV, during oral sex on a female and during analingus on any gender. It is placed over a person's anus or over the clitoris and vulva when your lover goes down on you. The Sheer Glyde dam has been approved by the FDA especially for safer sex. Other brands include Glyde Lollyes and Lixx.

At times hard to find, dental dams can be purchased at select drugstores or at specialty sex shops, like Babeland and Good Vibrations. Businesses specializing in safer sex supplies, like Condomania, also carry dental dams in a variety of sizes. Many of these businesses offer confidential online shopping and shipping services for those longing to make discreet purchases. Certain sexual and reproductive health organizations, like Planned Parenthood, or your local Department of Health or campus student health services may also have them available for free.

If you have trouble finding dental dams, or are in immediate need of protection, there are a couple of around-the-house substitutes at your disposal. You can: 1) tear off a sheet of nonmicrowavable (since it's nonporous) plastic wrap for a thinner alternative or 2) using scissors, carefully cut off the tip of an nonlubed, "dry" latex condom, as well as the elastic band at the open end. You'll want to then cut across the length of the condom for a stretchable, rectangular barrier. Yet another option is to trim the fingers (but not the thumb) off of a powder-free latex glove and cut along the side opposite the thumb.

When using a dental dam, make sure you cover your lover's entire anal opening area, holding the edges firmly with your hands as you work away. To make your experience better, consider adding flavored lube to your side. To give your partner more sensations, add a few dabs of his favorite silicone- or water-based lube. When you've had your fun, be sure to throw the dental dam away; it should never be reused, shared, reversed, or transferred from the vagina to the anus and vice versa.

Latex Surgical Gloves

Whether you want to cover cuts on your hands or fingers, to avoid jagged fingernails or hangnails, or simply want a smooth touch, gloves can provide feel-good sensations as you're delivering oral. Plus, they make for easy clean up, enabling you and your lover to seamlessly transition into afterplay and cuddling without worrying about mess. Nonlatex polyurethane gloves are available for those with latex sensitivities or allergies.

Sex Savvy

Ask your lover how he defines *sex*. This is important to know, as definitions can impact what is understood in sharing your sexual histories, including virginity status, and potential sexual health risks, including those from oral sexual activity.

Finger Cots

Found at your local pharmacy, these singular finger condoms are meant to protect fingers with cuts, allowing you to play with all sorts of parts while feeding your oral appetite.

But no matter what your choice of protection, the key to avoiding infection is to use prophylactics consistently and correctly. Latex offers the best protection, while polyurethane products are a great second choice for those with latex allergies. In any case, a non–animal-skin barrier should be used.

Talk about Your Sexual Health

Annually, 19 million Americans acquire an STD, which means that, sooner or later, you may have good reason to talk about your sexual health and safer sex with your lover. These discussions aren't easy, and if you're the one with an STD, you risk rejection, loss of confidentiality, potential humiliation, and other adverse consequences. Thankfully, there are ways you can prepare yourself for the tough conversation:

Get Informed

Knowledge is power, so become familiar with everything there is to know about STDs and safer sex. Educating yourself allows for greater understanding, ultimately reducing fears and giving you a sense of self and body ownership as you regain a sense of control and the power to cope. This also prepares you to correct any myths or calm any fears your lover may have.

Know Your Body

If you're infected with a viral STD, note when your outbreaks occur to better understand their timing. This might be when you're under a great deal of stress or drinking lots of caffeine. This will give you a greater sense of control over the infection and bodily changes, plus have you better able to counter triggers in taking better care of yourself and the best times to be sexually intimate.

Confide in a Professional

If you're distraught about your sexual health status or the risks involved in being intimate, talk to a mental health counselor. You may also want to find an online support group for others dealing with the same STD, as, rest assured, there are plenty of people in the same shoes.

Move the Conversation Forward

By successfully, confidently having sexual health discussions, be sure that they take place in an emotionally neutral environment and not when you're feeling horny and want to get all over your lover. Don't make a big deal out of them. This begins by not sounding anxious, panicky, or stressed, but rather seeking to sound calm and confident. You may also want to point out that STDs tend to get a bad rap. Oral herpes, genital herpes, shingles, and chicken pox, for example, are all due to having acquired a virus that remains in one's nervous system permanently. Yet genital herpes is stigmatized much more often than your common cold sore or chicken pox outbreak because it's related to sex.

In moving the conversation forward, be open-minded and ask that your partner do the same. Discuss your levels of comfort with STDs and safer sex, weighing the risks in light of your relationship, values, and what's important to you in a sexual relationship.

Suggest that you put your heads together in crafting a game plan on how you'll protect yourselves from here on out, or at least initially.

Some lovers may want to weigh the pros and cons of unprotected sex differently when in a long-term relationship, as some may be more willing to take or accept the risks involved in becoming more serious and intimate. In any case, tons of communication, trust, care, and protection are needed.

Talking isn't easy, but the benefits to your health and relationship are well worth it. Ultimately, you and your lover can feel closer in better knowing each other, and in becoming a team, protecting yourselves from here on out.

Sex Q & A

What STDs are detectable even if you don't show any symptoms?

Both men and women can be tested for HIV, syphilis, chlamydia, and gonorrhea. Gonorrhea and chlamydia screening involves a urine test or swab of the inside of a female's cervix or the swab of the inside of the penis. Doctors test for syphilis using a blood sample or swab from a genital sore, if present. Unfortunately, there is no screening test available for men in checking for HPV and no good screening test exists for either you or your guy for herpes, though blisters or ulcers can be scraped for tissue samples. Blood tests are available for herpes, but may be inconclusive. Be sure to ask for STD testing specifically, as different doctors have their own agenda during a gynecological exam and may not test for everything.

| Deciding Your Oral Sex Rules

New and different sexual relationships and opportunities require a constant re-evaluation of your sexual health, and just how much you want to or need to protect it. Ultimately, your sexual health comes down to your knowledge, skills, and motivation in protecting yourself. In becoming more informed, you learn more about your choices. You can do what's best for you given how much you're willing to roll the dice— or not.

So take the time to assess your levels of risk and decide upon the rules that will guide your oral sex efforts. You may, for example, always require a barrier method when having oral sex with somebody you just met. You may require that a partner get tested before having unprotected oral sex. This is a game where you draft your own guidelines, and hopefully have a partner who is on the same page. However, no matter how much you need to protect yourself, you still want to have fun too. Read on to find out how.

CHAPTER 11

Maximizing Your Orgasmic Potential

When it comes to sexual intimacy, nothing is quite as coveted as having an orgasm. Lovers spend a lot of time experimenting with different ways to reach climax, playing with the various hot spots sprinkled on or inside the body. With no two orgasmic experiences alike, you can elicit all sorts of climaxes and other reactions from one sex session to the next. How to maximize these during oral sex only adds to the infatuation lovers have with the pleasures had during such intimate exchanges.

Oral Sex Orgasms

Stimulating your man's genitals with your mouth is an incredibly effective way to bring him to climax. Oral sex allows for direct and easy stimulation of some of the body's prime hot spots, made even better in making them warm and wet. Getting head can result in some of the most powerful, wonderful orgasms ever experienced by your guy.

For some men (and women), sexual response induced from oral sex may result in multiple orgasms. Such a climactic response may present itself generally in any of the following ways:

1. Compound single orgasm. Each climax occurs separately, with your guy going back to a semi-aroused state between these peak responses. In this scenario, your lover will likely have his second orgasm a half an hour later.
2. Sequential multiple orgasms. Involves a series of climaxes that happen anywhere from two to ten minutes apart. Re-stimulation may be necessary.
3. Serial multiple orgasms. These orgasms occur in succession, with one right after the other. They may be separated by seconds. In other cases, these orgasms can feel like one huge, long orgasm. In either case, your lover may feel as though he is riding wave after wave of pleasure.

One of the ways your guy can experience an orgasm or multiple orgasms during oral sex is based on your ability to maintain a steady, constant rhythm when it comes to the action. In some cases, more pressure or a faster pace may be necessary. In any case, you'll need to maintain action to see your man's response through to orgasm.

Simultaneous Orgasms

Simultaneous orgasm is where you and your lover experience climax at the same time. While this can take place at any point during oral sex, depending on how *you* are being stimulated (including mentally), realizing simultaneous orgasm is often desired during 69 (see Chapter 3 for details). Engaging in *soixante-neuf* can elicit orgasm at the same time for lovers, provided that their sexual response states are in-sync.

While fun, lovers should be wary and not make simultaneous orgasm the goal of sex since it tends to be the exception to the rule. It's also quite sweet and sensuous to see a lover climax instead of necessarily being caught up in your own at the exact same time.

Rolls Off the Tongue

"We get lucky with simultaneous orgasm on occasion during 69, but in some ways it's more fun to take turns. It can be hard to really enjoy your own orgasm and somebody else's at the same time, so we tend not to make it our focus." }Frederick

Sex Savvy

When it comes to fellatio and pregnancy, Dutch research found that swallowing sperm during oral sex is correlated with diminished occurrence of pre-eclampsia. Another Australian study further found that pregnant women who perform oral sex on the father of their baby have safer, more successful pregnancies. Researchers believe that regular exposure to antigens in her partner's sperm helps a woman's immune system to more readily accept the baby.

Incorporating Other Hot Spots

While penile stimulation certainly makes for orgasmic reactions during oral sex, playing with other hot spots in addition to the oral action can make for different types of orgasms or multiple orgasms. Some of these additional hot spots include:

His Prostate

Found just under the bladder and behind the pubic bone, the male's prostate is a gland that can result in a great deal of pleasure when stimulated effectively. Approximately the size of a chestnut, this mass of muscle and glandular and connective tissue is the source of his physical orgasm, sending powerful, throbbing sensations throughout his pelvic region. While playing with this area can trigger a prostate-induced orgasm, firmly pressing on it via the perineum can also help a man to maintain his erection for longer sex sessions.

Sex Savvy

A man should empty his bladder prior to direct prostate play. If either of you are concerned about cleanliness, take a shower, perhaps using an anal douche kit if desired. Have towels and handwipes available, if needed, during sex play. Be sure to wash your hands right after you've finished fooling around.

Many lovers get off on the taboo nature of sex sessions that involve anal play—prostate stimulation included. Men who adore prostate play report that their orgasms become much more total body experiences, with these reactions deeper, longer-lasting, and more implosive, with ejaculation emitted as more of a spurt than a steady stream. Prostate stimulation can also help a man to experience multiple orgasms or a blended orgasm when the penis is stimulated at the same time.

In playing with his prostate, be sure that your partner is relaxed and fully aroused or well on his way there. Otherwise, stimulating this area could be uncomfortable, even painful. Using a glove (if not, make sure that your nails are trimmed and hangnail-free) and plenty of lubricant, slowly work your index or middle finger into his rectum. Once you're two to three inches up, press toward the stomach-side wall of the rectum. You'll feel a firm, round gland. Massage this area gently and slowly, becoming firmer in your pressure and rhythm as he gets more warmed up. Be sure to regularly ask him if your efforts feel good or not. If he has trouble relaxing, hold your finger against his prostate for ten to thirty seconds as he breathes deeply, or move your finger in and out of the anus in a light thrusting motion.

Once you're both comfortable with the movements, combine acts. Stimulate his prostate, massaging it, while performing fellatio. With experience, you'll be sliding or rocking your fingers rhythmically across his prostate in no time. Alternatively, you can thrust more than one finger in and out of his anus, pressing up against his prostate every time you go deep.

If at any point he loses his erection, don't freak out. Nothing is necessarily wrong. He may just need time to relax, especially if he's uncomfortable with prostate play. He may also need to focus more attention on his penis, since the prostate may have distracted him from his erection.

Perineum

For lovers not into prostate play via the rectum or for those looking into easier ways to stimulate the prostate during oral sex, stimulating the perineum is the way to go. This area of skin between a man's testicles and anus indirectly stimulates the prostate and penis when toyed with. To effectively stimulate, press up against this erogenous zone using the ball of your thumb. Feel for a slight indentation or ropy cord and, when stimulating the prostate, try caressing, tapping, massaging, or stroking the area with your tongue, fingertips, knuckle, or a sex toy like a vibrator. Experiment with different motions, rhythms, and directions, e.g., going clockwise, then counterclockwise.

His Butt

For a number of people, the bum is a hot spot in and of itself. He may just love having you grab, spank, or pull on his buns as you take him deeper. You can also massage or grip his butt cheeks while giving head, pinching or digging your nails into them in letting him know how turned on you are. Taking hold of his bum also allows you to better direct the angle, speed, and depth of the action—so don't be afraid to take charge!

Regardless of what you choose to do, the result will be a ripple effect throughout his loins, with his nerve endings in full effect from the tickling or light stinging you've managed. His scrotum will also come alive, wanting to get in on playtime. Make these areas ache even more in toying with his butt crack, running your fingers (or tongue during analingus) up and down the crease for greater stimulation. To give your fingers more of a gliding movement, use some lube.

His Anus

Even if your guy isn't into anal penetration of any sort, that's not to say that he may not be up for a little action around the anal opening. The anal opening is an area that's full of sensitive—and responsive—nerve endings that fire up when he becomes sexually excited. This area may come to life as more blood fills the area, making him more aroused and sensitive to your efforts. Even if he doesn't find himself particularly responsive to any stimulation in his backdoor area, he may simply get off on the taboo element of it. A number of people enjoy anal play of all sorts simply because they're treading on forbidden grounds. The thrill of doing something supposedly wrong, dirty, or downright taboo is what gets them going more than anything.

When it comes to anal play keep in mind that the area needs to be seduced; you don't want to rush in, rather a little bit of foreplay is necessary for anal play to be fully enjoyed. Most lovers don't like to be taken by surprise, so slowly work your fingers or tongue to the area. Analingus is one leisurely way to warm up his engines, slowly working your way to French kissing the area for his enjoyment.

| Tips for Maximizing His Orgasmic Response

Sometimes you may want to further intensify sex sessions. Other times, you may need to employ a few tricks in evoking more of an orgasmic response, especially during hot spot play that isn't working the way you want it to. In inviting more of a reaction, try the following . . .

Have Him Get out of His Head

Explain to your partner that he doesn't always need to be in control. Instead of resisting his sexual response, he should just relax, giving into sensations and the joy of being pleasured. He needs to get into the same head space that he would when going in for a deep tissue massage. He's here to take care of himself, let you do the work for him, and not think, but enjoy and lose himself in the feel-good sensations!

Encourage Him to Get Active

Sometimes your guy needs to move and get into the action, especially when oral starts to feel divine. So have him get his pelvis moving. Encourage him to squeeze his pelvic floor muscles rhythmically with

,ue movements or the sucking or thrusting action. Ask him to
.e hot spots that you're unable to attend to. While sometimes
i.   .e to lay there, other times he may need to get more physically
responsive.

Fantasize

Give your lover your blessing to lose himself in a favorite fantasy or
pretend that the situation is slightly different than what it is. This may
be imaging that you are his favorite movie star. He may be envisioning
that he's the star of a sold-out sex show. He needs to think about what
may be more desirable when it comes to the who (sorry, but it's often
so), what, when, where, and why for a completely different sexual situation that could throw him over the edge.

Get a Little Help

Whether either of you is tired, or he's not reacting in the way you
hoped, whip out a vibrator and let it do all of the work. After all, these
toys are there to enhance, help you out, and bring on reactions otherwise oft unattainable.

Start Him on a Kegel Regimen

Known collectively as the *pubbococcygeus muscle* (PC muscle), the
pelvic floor muscles allow lovers to have more control over their orgasmic responses. Learning to strengthen this muscle group with Kegel
exercises can make all of the difference in the world as pelvic floor
exercises can help him have better erections, a shorter recovery time
period, and a healthier prostate.

Kegel exercises can also help him to realize his multiorgasmic
potential as you give him head. This is in part because strengthen-
ing the area empowers him to delay and control orgasms. With stronger PCs, the intensity of his orgasms will increase quite a bit, and,

warning to you, his ejaculate is likelier to come out more forcefully and pleasurably.

To strengthen his PCs, instruct your guy to:

1. Identify his PC muscle group the next time he urinates by stopping his urine mid-stream.
2. To begin his PC regimen, he should slowly hold and release his PC muscle fifteen times, twice a day, focusing on his prostate, perineum, and anus.
3. Over time, have him gradually increase the number of reps to seventy-five repetitions, twice daily.
4. Once at seventy-five repetitions, he should move on to Phase II of these exercises, which involves holding each contraction for three counts instead of releasing immediately, then relaxing and repeating as many times as possible.
5. He should slowly work his way up to about fifty of these longer Kegels.

Your guy should see results in about a month. Once he feels as though he has good control of his PC muscle, encourage him to squeeze the area as you stimulate him orally. If easier, he may want to squeeze his muscles in rhythm with your movement. Have him keep doing so as both of you work to bring him to the "big O"!

Tease

While it's good to have great sexpectations, knowing what's going to happen can make for monotonous instead of moan-worthy action. So tease your lover, building sexual tension as you take him to the edge of bliss, only to attend to another hot spot. Keep coming back to his glans, but back off until neither you nor your lover can take it anymore. Then relish basking in a state of maximum sexual response.

Make Sure You Get Some Too!

Everybody has their own preferences when it comes to being giver or receiver and a major motive in giving for both sexes is the expectation that their partner will "return the favor." This expectation plays heavily in a person's willingness to go south of the border. Typically, women report feeling obliged to give head to partners after men go down on them. A woman's main motive to give head is to please her partner, but many women adore giving as much as they love to receive in return.

Rolls Off the Tongue

"I love both giving and receiving, but there's something about my partner becoming putty in my hands when I'm the one delivering. When I love and care about the person, it's so gratifying to know that they're feeling good and that my tongue and lips were the main cause for that!"

}Richard

Ideally, when it comes to oral sex, there are times you want to give, and then there are times you want to receive. And research shows that people are fairly good at taking turns, with 77 percent of men and 68 percent of women having given oral sex to a partner, and 79 percent of men and 73 percent of women having received oral sex from a partner. Mutual enthusiasm for receiving oral can have lovers in a quandary over who gets to be tonight's dessert. This can be a bit of a delicate matter if you've been so generous in your giving and practice of the techniques outlined in this book. Just remember, you deserve the opportunity to rest and receive after all your hard, loving labor.

Rolls Off the Tongue

"I can honestly say I have never had a bad oral sex experience, whether giving or receiving. I truly enjoy giving my partner oral pleasure. Typically, it enhances her ability to orgasm." }Neal

The best types of oral sexual experiences involve mutual pleasuring. While one sex session doesn't have to involve each partner receiving, lovers in healthy relationships tend to make sure that each has their time in the limelight. This is regardless of one's level of enthusiasm for wanting to give, or not. After all, in wanting to make a lover happy it's better to give than to receive.

Obviously, you're a giver. You just read an entire book on how to give your lover some of the best oral sex ever. If being a pleaser is in your nature, especially when it comes to sexual exchanges, it can be hard to let your lover do all of the work. But rest assured, he's likely more than willing to let you have your turn. After all, it is sometimes better to give than to receive and by allowing your lover to take a turn, you actually allow him to feel pleasure in pleasing you.

Sex Savvy

One 2003 study looking at the association between pleasure, sexual activities, and level of experience performing these activities found that that increased pleasure was associated with vaginal intercourse, receiving oral sex, and being masturbated by one's partner. Increased pleasure was also associated with more sexual activity and more sexual partners.

So give yourself permission to relax and be receptive. Mutual pleasuring is a must for a thriving, satisfying sex life, and your ability to invite such will make oral sex better for both of you—no matter your role.

APPENDIX A

Glossary

69 see "Sixty-Nine."

Afterplay post-sex touch and play.

Anal Beads plastic or latex beads strung together on a nylon or cotton cord that are used for anal sex play.

Anal Intercourse a sexual behavior involving insertion of one person's penis into another's anus.

Analingus stimulation of the anus with the mouth.

Anus the rectal opening located between the buttocks.

Butt Plug a dildo specially designed for anal and rectal pleasure via insertion into the anus.

Cock Ring a rubber, metal, or leather band worn around the base of the penis for sex play.

Condom a latex, polyurethane, or sheep skin, disposable sheath placed over an erect penis, which acts like a barrier to prevent pregnancy and the spread of STIs and HIV.

Corona raised ridge separating the glans from the body of penis; most sexually excitable region of penis.

Cunnilingus stimulation of the female genitals with the mouth.

Dental Dams latex or plastic wrap barriers placed over the vagina or anus during sexual activity to prevent the spread of STIs.

Dildo an artificial penis made of rubber, silicone, or latex.

Fellatio stimulation of the male genitals with the mouth.

Female Condom a disposable, polyurethane contraceptive tube, with a plastic ring at each end, that is inserted into the vagina to prevent pregnancy and the transmission of STIs and HIV.

Foreskin in uncircumcised males, the layer of skin covering the glans that retracts when the male is aroused and erect.

Frenulum tiny band of skin near the indentation on the underside of penis where the glans meets the shaft.

Glans in the male, the smooth, extremely sensitive tip (head) of the penis that contains numerous nerve endings; in the female, the extremely sensitive, visible external tip of the clitoris that protrudes like a small lump.

Multiple Orgasms a series of orgasmic responses that generally occur without dropping below the plateau level of arousal.

Oral Sex sexual activity involving mouth stimulation of the genitals.

Orgasm series of involuntary muscular contractions and a feeling of intense pleasure focused in the genitals that peak at sexual arousal and that may spread throughout the body; third and shortest phase of the sexual response cycle.

Penis the male reproductive and sex organ which passes sperm into the vagina and urine out of the body.

Perineum soft, hairless tissue between the genitals and anus in both sexes.

Polyurethane Condom plastic barrier, worn over an erect penis, that prevents pregnancy and the spread of STIs.

Rimming see "Analingus."

Safer Sex vaginal, anal, or oral sex involving practices that reduce the risk of pregnancy, HIV, and STIs.

Scrotum the pouch of skin, containing numerous sebaceous glands and hair, that holds the testicles.

Sexually Transmitted Disease (STD) see "Sexually Transmitted Infection."

Sexually Transmitted Infection (STI) any disease that can be transmitted via sexual contact.

Shaft in the male, the part of the penis that runs between the glans and root; in the female, the part of the clitoris that disappears into the body beneath the clitoral hood.

Sixty-Nine stimulation of the genitals with the mouths by both partners at the same time.

Soixante-Neuf see "Sixty-Nine."

STD see "Sexually Transmitted Disease."

STI see "Sexually Transmitted Infection."

Urethral Opening an acorn-shaped protrusion found between the clitoris and vaginal opening.

Vibrator a battery-operated or electric device that vibrates to stimulate body parts, particularly the genitals.

APPENDIX B
Resources

Internet Resources

American Social Health Association
www.ashastd.org
Offers sexual health information, particularly on sexually transmitted infections.

Centers for Disease Control and Prevention
www.cdc.gov
Presents sexual and reproductive health information. Oral sex and HIV risk information can be found at: *www.cdc.gov/hiv/resources/factsheets/pdf/oralsex.pdf*

Go Ask Alice!
www.goaskalice.columbia.edu
Columbia University's Health Education Program; Q&A site

Sexuality Information & Education Council of the United States
www.siecus.org
Nonprofit organization providing sex education programs and
materials

Sexuality Source, Inc.
www.sexualitysource.com (or www.yvonnekfulbright.com)
Offers sex education and consulting services, plus sex coaching and
information at *www.sensualfusion.com*

| Additional Reading

Fantasy

Advanced Sexual Fantasies. (DVD). (Sinclair).
The Erotic Guide to Sexual Fantasies for Lovers. (DVD). (Sinclair).

Kama Sutra

The Better Sex Guide to the Kama Sutra Set. (DVD). (Sinclair). 2004.

Sex Communication

Fulbright, Yvonne K. *Sultry Sex Talk to Seduce Any Lover: Lust-
Inducing Lingo and Titillating Tactics for Maximizing Your Pleasure*.
(Quiver, 2010). Beverly, MA.

Sex Therapy

American Association of Sex Educators, Counselors & Therapists
www.aasect.org

Society for Sex Therapy & Research
www.sstarnet.org

Sex Toys/Sexual Enhancements (mail order sexual enhancers, books, and DVDs)

Babeland
www.babeland.com

Sinclair Intimacy Institute
www.sinclair.com

Sexual Health

Fulbright, Yvonne K. *The Hot Guide to Safer Sex*. (Hunter House, 2003). Alamda, CA.

Planned Parenthood Federation of America
www.ppfa.org

Sexual Health Network
www.sexualhealth.com
Provides sexuality information, education and other resources

Sexual Pleasuring

Fulbright, Yvonne K. *The Better Sex Guide to Extraordinary Lovemaking*. (Quiver, 2010). Beverly, MA.

Fulbright, Yvonne K. *Pleasuring: The Secrets to Sexual Satisfaction*. (Hollan, 2008). Beverly, MA.

Fulbright, Yvonne K. *Touch Me There! A Hands-On Guide to Your Orgasmic Hot Spots*. (Hunter House, 2005). Alameda, CA.

McCarthy, Barry W. and Michael E Metz. *Men's Sexual Health: Fitness for Satisfying Sex*. (Routledge, 2008). New York, NY.

Stewart, Jessica. *The Complete Manual of Sexual Positions*. (Sexual Enrichment Series).Chatsworth, CA.

Tantric Sex

Anand, Margo. *The Art of Sexual Ecstasy*. (Putnam, 1989). New York, NY.

Lacroix, Nitya. *The Art of Tantric Sex*. (DK, 1997). New York, NY.

Sarita, Ma Ananda and Swami Anand Geho. *Tantric Love*. (Fireside, 2001). New York, NY.

Schulte, Christa. *Tantric Sex for Women*. (Hunter House, 2005). Alameda, CA.

Oral Sex Instruction DVDs

Better Sex Video Series: The Art of Oral Loving. (DVD). (Sinclair). 2006.

The Expert Guide to Oral Sex Part II: Fellatio. (DVD). (Tristan Taormino). Vivid.

Nina Hartley's Advanced Guide to Oral Sex. (DVD). Adam & Eve. 1998.

Index

Note: Page numbers in *italics* include illustrations.

playfulness in, 52
role-playing and, 53–55
Foreskin, *14*, 15, 60, 114–15
Frenulum, *14*, 16, 62, 75
From-behind position, 32–33
Furniture, erotic, 39–40

Gagging, 40, 63, 95–97, 98, 120
Genital warts, 133
Giving head. *See* Fellatio
Glans, *14*, 15, 53, 60, 62, 65
"Glory holes," 9
Glossary, 161–64
Go Deep Oral Sex Mints, 95
Go Deep Oral Spray, 95
Going down, 11, 55. *See also* Fellatio
Gonorrhea, 133, 144
Guilt, 94–95

Handcuffs, 44
Hands, 51, 63–64, 77
Head Candy, 97
Health benefits, 106–7
Hepatitis, 133, 134
Herpes, 133, 137, 138, 144
History of Fellatio (Leguay), 9
HIV (human immunodeficiency
  virus), 133, 135, 139, 144
Homosexuality, 135
Hormones, 17, 18, 46
Hot spots. *See also* Erogenous zones
  anus as, 152–53
  butt as, 152
  ignoring, 91
  inner, 17–18
  outer, 15–17
  perineum and, 151–52

prostate as, 150–51
tongue flutters on, 65
HPV (anal warts), 132, 134, 138
Humming, 66

Intercourse, 44
Intimacy, 9–10, 104, 107

Jaw fatigue, 97–98
Jeremy, Ron, 112
Jolie, Angelina, 48

Kakila. See 69 Positions
Kama Sutra
  history of, 83
  kissing and, 83
  69 position in, *87*
  techniques, 83, 84–85, 86
Kegel exercises, 100, 154–55
Kinsey Institute for Sex, Gender &
  Reproduction, 110
Kissing
  after orgasm, 106
  during afterplay, 66
  Amrachushita technique in, 86
  Chumbitaka technique in, 86
  as coreplay, 47–48
  as foreplay, 44–49
  groin, 60
  increasing hormones, 46
  Kama Sutra and, 83
  lingam, 84–86
  lip care and, 48–49
  lip sticks and, 49
  role of, 45–46
  styles, 47
Knees, 28–*29*, 91

About the Author

Yvonne K. Fulbright, PhD—sexologist, author, relationship expert, advice columnist, and television and radio personality—has been featured in hundreds of media outlets around the globe, including *The Tyra Banks Show,* NBC's *Today* show, *USA Today,* the *New York Times, Cosmopolitan,* and the Austrian Broadcasting Company. Fulbright received her master's degree in human sexuality education from the University of Pennsylvania and her PhD in International Community Health Education, focusing on sexual health, from New York University. She is currently a professor at both American University and Argosy University, a member of the Sinclair Advisory Council the sex columnist for *Cosmopolitan*, and Iceland's *Morgunbladid* and sexual health and relationship ambassador for Astroglide. She blogs for Huffingtonpost.com and is the sex expert for several media outlets including Comcast's "Dating on Demand" squad, SexHealthGuru.com, and the syndicated radio show *Your Time with Kim Iverson.* She is a Certified Sex Educator through the American Association of Sex Educators, Counselors, and Therapists (AASECT), where she provides editorial direction for *Contemporary Sexuality.* Yvonne currently lives in Washington, DC, where she runs Sensualfusion.com. For more information on Yvonne, visit *www.sexuality source.com.*

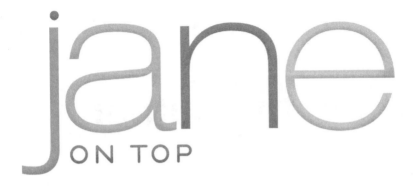